Successful Hypnotherapy

An insight into all aspects of the hypnotherapist's profession, giving clear guidance on learning the art of hypnosis and its practice

Successful Hypnotherapy

by

Neil French

THORSONS

THORSONS PUBLISHERS LIMITED
Wellingborough, Northamptonshire

First published 1984

British Library Cataloguing in Publication Data

French, Neil
Successful hypnotherapy.
1. Hypnotism — Therapeutic use
I. Title
615.8′512 RC495

ISBN 0-7225-0911-1

Printed and bound in Great Britain

CONTENTS

INTRODUCTION

Have you seen those notices in busy shops and offices which read: 'The impossible performed immediately – miracles take a little longer'? Well, I feel rather as though I am attempting something like that at the moment. Having discarded at least a hundred opening paragraphs for this book, I have decided simply to explain my predicament and hope you will understand.

What I want to say in the pages that follow ought to be of interest to every man, woman and child; because that is who it is about. The subject is fascinating for many reasons – not the least of which is that it is about ourselves. But, if I do not watch my step it will get labelled as just another boring book on psychology. Believe me, it is not.

The foregoing has prompted me to write the book in an unusual way, the better to capture and keep your interest, and the way I have decided upon is to write as though you, the reader, had asked me how to become a hypnotherapist and psychoanalyst. That is what I am by the way; a hypnotherapist and a psychoanalyst, which can be abbreviated to the title hypno-analyst.

I should think, by the time you have finished, you will probably decide you would prefer to sell snowballs in the middle of the Sahara, rather than choose my occupation. But I hope, for your own sake, that you have not just picked up the book out of idle curiosity, because soon it is certain to capture your attention, and one or two of its truths are going to strike to the very core of your civilized veneer.

1.
THE PRACTITIONER

When asked to say what words in the English language one would associate most with the occupation of doctor, the general sort of replies would be: clever, professional, helpful, trained, etc.; a salesman would rate: glib, aggressive, pushing, smart, etc.; and a tycoon would fare no worse than: ruthless, successful, powerful, etc. But now try the word hypnotist, and immediately: charlatan, faker, black magic, etc., spring to mind. A maligned subject, hypnosis has certainly achieved more than its fair share of notoriety. Since 1770, when Franz Anton Mesmer, whose name lives on in the English language as mesmerism, was first decried by traditional medicine, a long succession of other supposed charlatans have continued to use hypnosis to transform the lives of countless thousands of sufferers through the ages.

There is nothing magical about hypnosis at all, so it follows that there can be nothing magical about any cure or relief it helps create – in fact, hypnosis is a perfectly natural phenomenon occurring in man and animals, and is as much a part of our functioning, as are seeing and hearing.

Anyone who has experienced the hypnotic state at first hand will most likely say: 'It didn't work for me, I never went under.' In fact the state closely resembles our normal awareness. Far from being asleep as is popularly supposed, it is, if anything, a state of heightened awareness, at one with a feeling of calm and lethargic relaxation, and it is inconceivable that anyone could come to harm as a result of it.

Why then the tarnished image? The answer must of course lie in ignorance. In olden days, anything not understood was feared, and despite our present-day enlightenment, old myths die hard. The medical profession is totally committed to a multi-million-pound industry of drug therapy, and is desperately short of the one thing that is vital to any therapy involving hypnosis, and that is 'time'.

Although it would seem a barbarous act of self-interest on the part of traditional medicine totally to reject techniques which hold such potential for the relief of suffering in mankind, it should be appreciated that our modern-day acceptance of a subconscious mind and its part in our functioning was certainly not an acceptance years ago. Any symptoms created by an action of the subconscious were likely to be dismissed as unexplainable, or perhaps as evil spirits. Any cure from them had to be miraculous, or black magic. For these reasons, then and later, medicine ignored a priceless technique for the improvement of the human lot.

It has to be appreciated that hypnosis is not a treatment in itself, but is only an aid to other therapy, and, whereas it is very pleasant and relaxing to enter the hypnotic state for a while, merely to do so serves no lasting purpose. It is what takes place when experiencing the state that matters, and this is probably the biggest single reason for any objection to it. A good hypnotist is not necessarily a good therapist, and one sometimes hears people say: 'I went to a hypnotist but "it" didn't work for me.' If there is to be a benefit to the person, then the hypnotist needs to have the skill of a general practitioner, the knowlege of a psychoanalyst, the forebearance of a clergyman, the intuition of a detective and a moral ethic of the highest order. As he can shape and improve the whole lives of those he treats, he must be free himself from any 'hang-ups' which may affect his own judgement. To say that such men, or women, do not grow on trees is to understate the obvious. Indeed, it is regrettable, but true, that hypnotherapy can attract to its ranks those who themselves need help, and unknowingly are subconsciously seeking a relief from inner anxiety.

I really would like you to assume, all the time you are reading this book, that you actually are studying to be a hypnotherapist; I promise it will make far more interesting reading. The book, being a progressive build-up of information, may well give the impression that some of the earlier material seems contentious, but I am willing to bet that you will not think that by the last page. During the early parts it will be helpful to your overall final depth of understanding if you try to avoid negatives in your own thoughts, such as 'there could be a different explanation of that'. Try at first to absorb without criticism and then do your criticizing with the advantage of hindsight.

Hypnosis itself is comparatively easy to learn and if you have an interest in the subject you may well be disappointed at how long it takes me to get around to elaborating fully upon the uses of it. Please be patient. It is common sense which says that a person usually drives a motor car somewhat better if he has an understanding of the engine, the clutch, the gearbox, and other such functions; and, likewise, just to be a hypnotist is not really to be anything. I always, inwardly, feel mildly insulted by the name hypnotist – whereas the terms hypnotherapist, psychotherapist, and psychoanalyst I find acceptable.

A hypnotherapist may, for all practical purposes, be defined as a practitioner who uses the power of suggestion to induce the hypnotic state in his client and then utilizes the altered state of awareness of the client to bring about a therapeutic end. This would normally be to assist the person to deal effectively with something which, hitherto, had been inside himself or herself, but outside his own control – usually to help him stop doing something that he does not want to do, or start doing something that he would like to be able to do.

Purists and theorists will likely haggle for decades over definitions of hypnosis itself (if indeed such a state really exists at all – perhaps, after all, there is only really suggestion itself). At a practical level it would be better to settle for a definition such as: 'A state of relaxation and concentration, at one with a state of heightened awareness, induced by suggestion; a non-addictive power for good, and a natural manifestation of the mind at work.' Most importantly, henceforward, please regard hypnosis and the induced state of hypnosis not as an end result but merely as a beginning to something else.

Supposing you asked a person, who in fact is a doctor, what his occupation is, and he replied, 'Oh, I'm a "medical profession".' Your puzzlement as to what he really meant by the improper use of the English language would lead you to ask what he was within the medical profession – say surgeon, or GP, or midwife. Really the same applies to the word 'hypnotherapist', which of course combines the use of hypnosis and therapy – Aha! but which therapy, you ask, since hypnosis itself is not a therapy at all. Well, I hope by the time I have finished you will see how critical your question really is.

A word about the student – the potential hypnotherapist/psychotherapist – even though you are only pretending you want to be one. Ample evidence exists that within the psychiatric profession there is a higher rate of suicide, a higher rate of alcoholism, and a higher rate of sexual malfunction than within any of the other professions which exist. Although separate figures are not available for psychotherapists and hypnotherapists, there is abundant reason to believe that the same facts hold good. The work manifestly attracts as practitioners people who are themselves in need of treatment. Plenty of these people would say that they were perfectly happy, that there was nothing wrong with them, and that therefore they had no need of treatment themselves. However, let us take as our first consideration not the therapist but the person he is going to treat. Is this untreated therapist really competent and will he truly deal with his client adequately? Could he be sure that:

1. not choosing to see unpalatable characteristics in himself, he may cause his clients to gloss over these characteristics?
2. he attributes his own unwanted characteristics to both his patients and/or colleagues?
3. he does not fully realize what his own client is going through?
4. feeling some of his own urges or desires to be wrong, he passes these criticisms to his clients?
5. feeling himself inferior and vulnerable (or feeling himself superior and dictatorial), he adopts an incorrect attitude towards his clients?
6. his judgement is, unknown to himself, distorted generally?
7. he has rationalized as appropriate inadequate – or no – treatment for himself, and perhaps too will consider inadequate treatment for his client?

Many, many practitioners will claim that they are an exception, that their mental health, insight and understanding is such that they have no need of treatment. But experience proves that the only practitioners who consistently and persistently get good results with clients, and who remain in private practice year upon year, are those who have entrusted their own 'hang-ups' to a competent therapist before ever embarking on practice themselves. As a student of hypnotherapy you are seeking to enter the world of 'alternative medicine' at a time when, as Ivan Illich, the Austrian educationist, said, 'Modern medicine has become a major threat to the nation's health, and its potential for social, even physical disruption, is rivalled only by the perils inherent in the industrialized production of food.' You would be well advised to heed 'man, know thyself'.

Jung was explicit when he stated that a therapist must know his own shadow and have had real experience of the unconscious forces he is now helping his client to face. He cannot evade his own difficulties by trying to cure other people; he must first cure himself or be cured. In sharing his patients' experiences he risks contamination by their illness, even as a doctor risks infection by physical illness, and he needs all the stability that self-knowledge can bring. This belief that nervous disorders are as transmissible as the common cold is not confined to Jung, and a well-documented phenomenon exists with the self-explanatory label 'Therapists burn up'.

Should you think that I am labouring this point, I will forewarn you; I will return to it again before we have finished, and perhaps you are already glad that you are only pretending that you want to learn to be a therapist.

THE THERAPIST and the BRITISH LAW

The titles hypnotherapist and psychotherapist, or indeed psychoanalyst, are not protected in law, the only prescribed titles being: chemist, chiropodist, dentist, dental surgeon, dental practitioner, dietician, doctor, druggist, general practitioner, medical laboratory technician, midwife, nurse, occupational therapist, optician, orthoptist, physiotherapist, pharmacist, radiographer, remedial gymnast, surgeon, veterinary surgeon, veterinary practitioner.

It is a criminal offence to use any of these specified titles unless the person is on the statutory register of the persons holding such qualifications. Even with non-specified titles such as ours, or estate agents, and valuers and the like, it would technically be an infringement of the law to use the title unless you were capable of carrying out the actions the title suggests. Should you wish to call yourelf an estate agent and valuer you would first have to be able to offer houses etc., for sale and to be able to arrive at a realistic estimate of their true value.

Generally speaking, British law is more helpful to alternative medicine than, for example, American law, but that does not mean to infer that a practitioner is totally uncontrolled. Naturally he is subject to laws such as the Trades Description Act and so on. Also he has a duty of care to his client, the breach of which would be professional negligence.

Negligence, expressed in general terms, is the 'duty of care' that one person is required to have for another person in their dealings or contacts with them. A therapist has a 'duty of care' towards his clients and if he fails to exercise that duty diligently then he exposes himself to the risk of a claim for punitive damages to redress the 'tort', or wrong, he has done the person. In order to ensure that the 'duty of care' imposed on the therapist is realistic and not beyond his skills and knowledge, it is obviously necessary to make sure that the client has not been misinformed as to what is or is not possible and likely by the actions of the therapist. It is essential to ensure that the therapist does not claim, even by implication, that he has the same knowledge, skills and procedures as are contained within established medicine. A therapist would be wrong to undertake a case where he lacked the necessary skills and knowledge to treat it, as he would equally be wrong by incorrectly applying such skills and knowledge as he had. Probably the most important 'duty of care' the therapist has towards his client is that where he knows or, in the opinion of a reasonable man, ought to have known, that the particular case was outside the province of his particular skills, then he has a duty to tell the person so and to take active measures to correct the situation by referring the person to somebody else or summoning additional skills to assist.

British law requires that if, at the time of death the deceased had not consulted a doctor during the preceding month, a post-mortem examination must be performed – frequently leading to an inquest. As well as people who are gravely ill, those who are terminally ill and people who are suicidal also consult therapists, and the therapist should be always alert to the possibility of a death occurring between consultations. Ensure that such people do see their doctors at a maximum of four-weekly intervals; then, should death occur, there is every hope that a certificate would be issued and an inquest avoided. The last thing any therapist wants is criticism at an inquest to the effect that his 'lay' treatment accelerated the person's demise. Your name in the newspapers you want, your name in the Sunday rags you do not want!

Professional indemnity insurance is a must, and, in the author's opinion, it would be bordering on the criminally negligent to practise without such cover. Amounts of monetary redress awarded by courts in cases of civil tort are increasing enormously, and legal costs are horrific. In fact, it would be fair to say that even defending an action where the therapist is in the right would probably bring the average practitioner to his financial knees.

In common with many self-employed people, hypnotherapists often practise from their own homes. The pitfalls of home practice need consideration. Firstly, the legal aspect: Should the establishment of a private practice constitute a 'material change of use' from purely residential to mixed residential and business, then planning consent is required and unauthorized use can produce substantial fines. Now, exactly what a 'material change' is lacks an accurate interpretation, but planning departments take into account whether the room(s) is going to serve a dual purpose, the amount of work actually done in the home, the number of people likely to be visiting, and so on. It had been ruled that doctors and dentists can use their own home for consulting rooms, and presumably the same professional category would be extended to hypnotherapists, but it has equally been ruled that if they take a partner, or take into employment a secretary, or indeed any employee, then planning permission is required. Should you enquire from your local authority they are almost certain to ask you to submit an application 'to clarify the point', and it is true to say that most local authorities refuse applications put before them for fear of setting too much of a precedent. Again it would be fair to say that the local authority would only become involved if you approached them yourself, or if somebody else complained about you. Should the local authority investigate and decide an unauthorized change of use has occurred they will serve an enforcement notice requesting a cessation, which would allow reasonable time to comply. Only then does the offender invoke the possibility of that £1000 fine and £50 daily penalty, and then only after he has been given an opportunity to appeal to the Department of the Environment. Rates would normally only be increased to business rates if the room(s) had been set aside entirely for the business and was no longer used for residential purposes.

Probably the main consideration in relation to practising from home is the intrusion into your own private life. Many people who visit a therapist are in the grip of a neurosis and justifiably deserve the title 'neurotic' (even if the non-technical, mildly slanderous, interpretation of that word is used). Do not expect neurotic people to abide by more socially acceptable standards of behaviour, and don't be too surprised if your phone, or front-door bell, goes at about 3 a.m. with a suicidal melancholic demanding an immediate, if not sooner, cure from his malaise. Perhaps the author should at this point admit that his own private phone is ex-directory, that he practises from lock-up consulting rooms away from his own residence, and parries any questions about his address as, 'oh, the other side of Bournemouth', which, whilst being strictly true, is vague enough to deter further questioning. One further point on this vexatious question: a therapist treats people from just about every walk of life. Nervous disorders do not discriminate against rich or poor, and people (being people) do tend to judge others by appearances. Should you live in a ten-bedroomed Georgian mansion your poorer clients are going to be impressed, or indeed in awe; should you live in a 'two-up and two-down' terraced, your wealthier clients are going to drive straight past. Perhaps, at the end of your treatment, neither sector would be so bigoted – but you have to make the initial contact. The author has often had clients say, 'It is difficult to visualize you away from these offices' and, to be honest, that is the way I prefer it. At a later stage we will be talking about the phenomenon of transference, when it would pay to recall this discussion about location of consulting rooms.

There is very little criminal law which specifically mentions hypnosis. The British Hypnotism Act of 1952 was primarily aimed at the control of stage performances, which to an extent it deals with quite effectively. Legislature of the time avoided the definition of hypnosis and merely stated:

> In the Act, hypnotism shall have the following meaning assigned to it, that is to say: hypnotism includes hypnotism, mesmerism, and any similar act or process which produces or is intended to produce in any person any form of induced sleep or trance in which the susceptibility of the mind of that person to suggestion or direction is increased, but does not include hypnotism, mesmerism or any such act or process which is self-induced.

Their description could be torn to shreds by modern understanding of the subject, but there again, I have seen a conference of professional users of hypnosis fall apart in disorder, and eventually break up, solely through trying to define 'hypnosis'. That is not our purpose anyway – we have a much more tortuous route to follow.

There have been other attempts in the UK to bring legislation to bear upon the subject of hypnotherapy and psychotherapy. As long ago as 1971 the Foster Committee reported to Parliament that the need for legislation existed, and as recently as 1981 an MP (Gerald Bright) tried to get a bill through to create a Council for Psychotherapy. No ethical practising psychotherapist need fear such legislation – firstly, because the chances of any reaching the statute-books in the next decade are extremely remote; and secondly, because any enactment would inevitably contain a 'grandfather clause' to allow existing practitioners to continue.

In the UK a therapist's advertising in the press is regulated by a code of advertising practice. Until 1982 the therapist's advertisements were required to be confined to the so-called 'visiting card' advertisement containing only such particulars as would normally be on a visiting card, e.g. name, address, qualifications, hours, etc. and any claims, or indication of problems assisted, were not allowed. The committee of the Code of Advertising Practice have relaxed their rule slightly to allow claims to assist smoking and slimming. Interpretation of these rules varies from newspaper to newspaper.

Assuming everything I have said so far has intrigued you sufficiently for you to want to know a little more about we humans (and remember, in the kingdom of the blind he with only one eye is king), let us now look into the human psyche.

2.
CHARACTER TYPES AND THEIR SYMPTOMS

In order to begin to understand people and their problems, you will first have to understand the very cornerstone of these writings: the ability of the human mind to *repress* unpleasantness.

> 'I did this,' says my memory.
> 'I cannot have done this,' says my pride . . . and remains inexorable.
> In the end – memory yields. (Nietzsche)

The whole process of repression is difficult to explain and even more difficult to understand. Unquestionably the best way to understand it is to have a repression released from yourself – for, believe me, you have undoubtedly got many within you. I do not want to get bogged down with technicalities of pre-conscious, sub-conscious, unconscious definitions, so throughout the book I will use the term subconscious. (I will also use the definitive 'he' throughout the book, hopefully assuming that all female readers will realize it is for expediency only and devoid of any chauvinistic ulterior motive.)

A person's mind will repress (with convenient amnesia) something very unpalatable to that person. Where the process is, for want of a better description, half-hearted, we will call it a disavowal. To illustrate this we need only describe the child who has been punished and sent to bed for naughtiness. Let us imagine the parent worrying for an hour or so over the severity of the punishment, finally relenting and going to the child's room to sympathize. Frequently the child would be happily playing with some new interest, the previous wrongdoing having been cheerfully disavowed. As it transpired, the only worrying over the issue had been done by the parent.

Let us now go a step further, and assume that the originating incident had created enormous emotion in the child, say, for instance, shame. The possibility now arises that the emotion is sufficient to penetrate the subconscious of the mind so that the whole incident becomes totally concealed from the normal intellectual awareness of the child. Not just a disavowal but a total repression. The child will become consciously unaware that the incident ever took place at all – and if questioned about it in later life would, on oath, deny that such an incident had ever occurred. Furthermore, he would firmly believe that he was speaking the truth.

The difference between a disavowal and a repression hinges upon the fact that in the disavowal the person knows the incident happened, but prefers not to think about it (rose-tinted spectacles if you like); in the case of the repression the person, quite genuinely, does not know that the incident ever occurred.

Should you have understood so far you are already a step ahead of the average psychiatrist who, often due to the internal resistance of his own repressions, does not like to believe in their existence, and even where he does believe, still thinks they are totally inaccessible, doing little harm, and that sleeping dogs are best left to lie. You are going to discover to the contrary. Please understand, I have not said that unpleasant, frightening, shameful and sad incidents will be repressed into the subconscious. I have only said that they may be repressed if the amount of emotion generated is sufficient.

A good example would be the road-accident victim who, quite truthfully, tells the police: 'I remember backing my car out of the drive, and I remember waking up in hospital, but of the drive to the scene of the accident, or the accident itself, I remember nothing.' His mind, to ensure that the awfulness of that jagged windscreen tearing his face apart has been repressed, has also effectively concealed the rest of the journey, and the ambulance ride too.

Although we will be returning to the subject of repression again, please accept at face value for the time being, that what I have written in true. This process happens in humans in their formative years; it also occasionally happens in female subjects during, or after, pregnancy. Indeed, like the illustration of the road accident, it can happen at any time that the emotion is strong enough and this process of repression has an effect upon the organism as a whole. What these effects can be, and the meaning for us as therapists, I will leave till later.

Let us continue with the more normal development pattern. To begin to understand people and their problems you have to look right back to their character formation; you need to learn how a person's behaviour pattern is learned, and the factors which influence its formation.

You have heard sayings like 'The hand that rocks the cradle rules the earth,' and 'Give me the child and I will show you the man.' These sayings do not exist without foundation. Our basic character, the way in which we react to, and deal with, the environment, is formed within us at a very early age.

The three main stages of human development are as follows:

1. The ORAL stage – from birth to about 2½–3 years.
2. The ANAL stage – from about 2½/3 years to about 5 years.
3. The GENITAL stage – from about 5 years to puberty.

Where the predominant character traits are formed in the first stage, we call the resultant personality Oral, or more accurately, 'pre-genital, oral group, schizoidal personality'.

Where the main character traits are not formed in the Oral period but develop in the Anal period, we call the resultant personality Anal, or more accurately, 'pre-genital, anal group, paranoidal or obsessional personality'.

Where the basic character remains unformed until the Genital period, we call the resultant personality Genital, or more accurately, 'genital group, hysterical personality'.

At this stage be reassured that the words, terms and descriptions I am using are common to most disciplines of psychology and psychiatry, although in many cases the words do not have necessarily the same meaning as their more customary day-to-day usage. Where differences exist, they are of small consequence; for example, some schools of psychology would call the second development period the sadistic period or anal/sadistic period. It matters not – we are aiming for a basic understanding of what makes us tick. The names for the three development stages are fairly self-explanatory. In our earliest years we experience everything orally – give a baby something, and it goes straight to the mouth. Then we come to the momentous step of bowel control with its attendant failures and successes, until we reach the curiosity stage of our own, and others' genitals, which eventually brings us to puberty and full sexual awareness. You are going to find that people are surprisingly, perhaps even pathetically, predictable and it is possible to 'brand' everyone as one of the three main types.

Look now at the three main types and see how many people you know (including yourself) who can be labelled quite neatly as a character type. Please remember, however, that no one person could conform to all the requirements of the character type. One does not expect to find all the symptoms and character traits in any one individual. It is the type, the motivation and the outlook which is so characteristic.

CHARACTER TYPES

We start with the more stable personality, the 'pre-genital, oral group of schizoidal personality'.

Basically shy people at heart. Rather retiring and introverted. Rather self-centred, but certainly not selfish. They tend to refer everything inwards to their own self, and because of this tend to be easily hurt and readily affected by the emotions of others. They give things an inner value that other people cannot see and, if anything, take things too seriously as a consequence. They include life's day-dreamers, and have an active fantasy life; always building up hopes, and over-reacting with depression to the anti-climax of harsh reality. They usually have a very good imagination and a natural talent of creativity, are quite often artistic in one or more of the many art forms, but just as often fail to find any means of liberating and expressing this art form within themselves. In their emotional life they are capable of great intensity of feeling, but it is seldom that they can find the words to express their feelings adequately. They have a good insight into the character of other people, but tend to see themselves as being misunderstood, as though there was a gap separating them from others. They are basically honest and have a regard for other people and their feelings; not the ones to use or exploit other people and therefore not obsessed by monetary gain or self-aggrandizement. They are somewhat over-sensitive, and nostalgic about the past. They are remarkably willing to see their own failings and tolerant of others, but the most noticeable characteristic is their mood swings – what is known as the 'all or nothing' reaction – switching in an instant from being happy and bright and cheerful to being depressed and forlorn. Look at the mood swings of a babe in arms and you see the predisposition of 'oral' folk. They carry that 'all or nothing' reaction to most aspects of their life.

Next let us look at the anal mentality, the pre-genital group of paranoidal or obsessional personality.

These are a power-seeking and very ruthless sort of people. Brooding and ruminative, jealous and suspicious, they often get ideas that others are plotting and planning against them (really only their own plots and schemes projected outwards). They tend to be very possessive, both with people and possessions – indeed, they regard people as pawns to be used and manipulated. They take pleasure in hurting others and will look for chinks in their armour to strike at weaknesses in order to make the suffering as great as possible; their unconscious motivation for this is that by so doing, by weakening another, one gains strength oneself (a bizarre form of vampirism). Obsessional traits predominate, such as routine, order, method, discipline, and the belief that might is right, and that the fit will survive. They are often extremely vain and egotistical, with a holier-than-thou attitude which says that everybody else is wrong and they are right. Boastful and self-seeking, they see themselves as the world's greatest actor, lover, author (whatever prevails at the moment). They are very selfish people who have scant, if any, regard for other people's feelings, and are usually very materialistic, bordering on meanness. Usually they have a bad temper and woe betide the person who opposes them. They consider their own insight perfect whereas in reality they have hardly any at all. Usually they demonstrate extremes (in either direction) of personal hygiene. The predominant and most noticeable feature is their brooding, ruminative sort of outlook on life. Although they are extremely adept at concealing their true nature beneath a veneer of charm and good manners, those who know them well can easily see beneath that suave exterior to the rather shallow character beneath.

Finally let us look at the third category, the late developers of life – the genital group of hysterical personality.

Very shallow people with very little, or no depth to their character at all. Extremely extroverted, always showing off, always hogging the limelight. The word that most describes them is 'actors'. They have no depth at all to their emotions or feelings, but go to great lengths to convince you of the contrary, by tremendous displays of affection, or of emotion. However well they do in life, they remain lacking in any inner life or any sort of insight, they are rather gullible and credible, and mentally immature. They are always showing off and acting out a part, demanding others' admiration – but as others can usually see straight through their shams and pretences, they seldom get any. Their favourite place would be the centre of attention at some fun occasion, sparkling like frothy champagne, witty and bright and monopolizing the scene. It never enters their head that others might not be impressed by their cavorting, or the finery of their feathers. They'll bluster and bluff their way through any situation, but watch them if the environment becomes harsh and unkind. Now you see the complete absence of depth to their characters – they see themselves as the victim, the one who has been abused and misled. They will have an unending list of scapegoats and excuses, and if all else fails they'll produce some physical symptoms for others to sympathize with in order to take attention away from their own failings. The hysterical personality will swear his love will endure for ever, and leave on the next train. He'll flatter you, lavish pseudo-affection and endless compliments, but underneath he's as empty as that bottle of champagne. He's an actor first, foremost and last and if he can impress you, he's happy.

So, that's our three basic character types. Remember, nobody could conform exactly to one 'type' – you will always find elements of each character type within any one person, but there will always be a predominant trait and disposition which enables you to label them. The basic content of a person's character is usually fairly easy to spot, and it is going to be important in your future therapy that you learn to assess and categorize people within a short while of meeting them.

SYMPTOMS

Perhaps you have noted the similarity of the type titles to the names of mental illnesses:

Schizoidal – schizophrenia.
Paranoidal – paranoia.
Hysterical – hysteria or hysterical dissociation.

As a rule of thumb we describe a person as mentally ill when he or she is suffering from a psychosis rather than a neurosis, explained in the simplest and most elementary terms as follows:

> The neurotic knows very well his own abnormal behaviour is unusual and would like to correct it. The psychotic considers his own abnormal behaviour to be perfectly normal and usual, and has no desire to correct it.

As a hypnotherapist/psychotherapist you will be dealing only with the neuroses, the first-stage nervous disorders, so we will pay no attention to true mental illness, except in passing to say that it is really just a tremendous exaggeration of the neurotic behaviour, and neurotic behaviour is really only an exaggeration of 'normal' behaviour. Think about this for a moment and you will realize that the psychotic who hugs his knees and head together in a corner with his face turned away from the world is really a tremendous exaggeration of the agoraphobic who doesn't like to leave the safety of his own home. Similarly, 'smearing' and eating of faeces is again a tremendous exaggeration of lesser habits observable on public-toilet walls and perpetrated by 'normal' people.

Returning to our basic character types: each type has its own likely behavioural problems. Think again of 'oral' folk and that 'all or nothing' reaction – suddenly depression and melancholia become more understandable. The 'nothing' has triumphed over the 'all'.

Depression (Melancholia)

Depression is a temporary and passing thing. Melancholia is the same thing but in a permanent state, which responds neither to the passing of time, nor to the change of circumstances.

Melancholia exaggerates depression, so that there is a loss of energy and desire, a withdrawal of interest from the business of living, a predisposition to tears, apathy, listlessness and despair. All processes are reduced to low level, sometimes loss of appetite and wasting, or total disinterest in appearance. The person is giving a splendid imitation of that forlorn, deserted, abandoned, neglected child of years ago. Sometimes the person is very restless and self-accusing, even attempting self-injury or suicide – then it is termed agitated melancholia. Here, though, we have to make a point of distinction. Imagine for a moment a woman demonstrating the symptoms I have just outlined. Imagine asking for an explanation of her behaviour and being told that her husband died a week ago. You really then have to accept, with the attitude of a reasonable person, that her behaviour is in fact explainable; that it does not deserve to be called a nervous disorder, and that in fact she is in mourning, called 'reactive depression' for our purposes. Now switch to the other extreme and imagine that, as an explanation, the woman tendered the fact that her husband had died *ten years ago.* Inevitably now you will come to the conclusion that the woman is suffering some unconscious conflict which is causing the symptoms; and the husband's ten-year-old death is only what is called 'erroneous association' (more of that later).

Please note from this that the severity of a problem has to be judged from two viewpoints: one, to assess the severity of the symptoms being exhibited; and the other, to assess the presence of, or the absence of, real and justifiable causes. It is strange, but nevertheless a fact, that an extremely neurotic person may go happily through life demonstrating little or no symptoms of behavioural disorder, whereas an apparently stable and rational person may break down completely. The former behaved so because life remained, thanks to the intervention of fate, remarkably kind to him, e.g. good job, good income, good wife, good children, good holidays and the latter because life became, thanks to the intervention of fate, remarkably cruel to him, e.g. no job, no money, divorce, wayward offspring and constant pressure.

We will leave depression for a while, having noted that it affects mostly oral folk and is, when pathogenic, a symptom of an internal, but subconscious, conflict within the psyche, and we will look instead at another behavioural problem that affects oral people.

Compulsions
(not to be confused with obsessions, which will be discussed later)

The sufferer finds himself in the grip of a compulsion to carry some task through to a conclusion, only to find that completion of the task brings neither satisfaction nor relief, and the compulsive activity is quickly replaced by another one, to which the same large amount of drive and energy is applied. The person gives every indication of remorselessly being driven (which indeed he is – albeit by an inner force of which he may be unaware). Should anybody else interfere with the compulsive activity he becomes very resentful and gets very anxious and irritable until allowed to resume the activity. Should he force himself to quit the compulsion there is an immediate reaction of depression. The predominant factor is an irrational and highly compulsive drive which the individual finds virtually impossible to forgo. Sometimes it is extremely useful socially, as it can be directed towards work or hobbies, but his neglect of other considerations in order to carry out the compulsive task tends to nullify such benefits. We don't have to be very clever to see here a clear example of that 'all or nothing' reaction of those nice oral people.

What of the not so nice anal types? Examine now their behavioural disorders and see the obvious differences.

Obsessions

At first it sounds as though we are talking about the oral compulsions, but don't let the similarity of the words deceive you. The obsessional is totally different. He starts off with a very energetic disposition, is very self-willed, has reasonable intellectual gifts, reaches a satisfactory level of ethical development, and exhibits a degree of over-conscientiousness in his behaviour. What a contradictory hotch-potch of character traits. The forms his obsessions take are innumerable, and may be obsessional actions or obsessional thought. He has suffered this from his early (anal) years and he's made displacements and exchanges by the hundred by the time he knocks at your door. He's replaced one foolish idea in his head

('I think I'm Jesus Christ – but I know I'm not', would be a severe example) with another foolish idea, somewhat milder; or he's replaced one foolish obsessional action (like washing his hands every 7¾ minutes – every 7 minutes wouldn't suffice) for another equally foolish obsessional action. Watch the child tread on every crack in the pavement to make sure he gets ice-cream for tea and you get some insight into the obsessional and his totally absurd magical beliefs. That's the punch line of obsession: 'absurd magical belief', and what's more, he knows it's absurd. He will share your opinion of his stupidity, but he cannot help himself. He surrenders himself to the foolish thought or hands himself over to the obsessional action, only reluctantly, and is obliged against his own will to brood, with that anal brooding, ruminative quality, over the action or thought as though it was a vitally important aspect of his life – not, as it really is, a matter of indifference to him. Even Freud, the father of psychology, was driven to state: 'Certainly this is a crazy illness, and if one did not see it before one every day, one could not bring oneself to believe in it.' More of paranoid obsessionals later, but for now accept that if you were paid only on results, and you only had obsessionals to deal with, then you'd better frame your holiday snaps because you wouldn't be taking many more.

Every bit as difficult to deal with is the other behavioural disorder of the anals.

Hypochondria

According to him, nobody ever before had such a severe ailment as he. As you listen to his woebegone account of how terrible his amazing symptoms are, as he shows with ill-concealed delight the amazing stitches from his latest dreadful experience, you can hardly fail to notice the note of pride creeping into his voice. What has happened, of course, is that the brooding ruminative traits of his nature have latched on to parts of the body which are supposed to be diseased. That obsessional trait shows itself, because he's certainly obsessed with his illness. Actually there is not the slightest thing wrong with him, but for him ever to realize that would be impossible and, indeed, the unkindest cut of all. He wants his symptoms. He wallows in his symptoms, he enjoys every tortured minute of his martyrdom, and to him his symptoms are as real as a broken leg would be to you. He's convinced himself so well that he can frequently convince doctors and specialists, and the NHS foots the bill for a totally unnecessary operation or sequence of operations. Watch him preen himself and his satisfaction is obvious. He's convinced it was the most difficult and dangerous operation of its type the surgeon had ever performed. I will not labour it any more, but the message is clear – this is a person with a proud preoccupation with a supposed malfunction.

Let us move on now to that third type, the hysteric, and examine their likely behaviour disorders.

Conversion Hysteria

In this process the anxiety within the mind is converted into a bodily symptom (no, it's not the same thing as hypochondria – bear with me for a moment). The hysteric no more knows he's doing it than does the hypochondriac, but, unlike the hypochondriac, the hysteric is blissfully unconcerned about his physical problems. He can demonstrate faithfully and accurately all the signs and symptoms of a cardiac arrest, and be as unconcerned as if he'd broken a fingernail. What he is trying to do, unconsciously of course, is get his own way. He produces dramatic symptoms, like the good actor he is, to dominate and coerce the environment and get his own way. About the worst thing anyone can do is give in to him, because flushed with success he will make greater and greater demands, and produce more and more exaggerated symptoms. Let those close to him ignore his outbursts – so his audience, so necessary to his actor's ego, is not watching – then his symptoms go too. They will come back, though, next time he wants to get his own way. I mentioned when describing basic hysterical personality that, if his environment becomes unkind, he wants a scapegoat and, if he can't find one, then the quick appearance of a bodily symptom will deter investigation of his own shortcomings.

Hysterical Dissociation

An amazing phenomenon of the mind, which is surprisingly more common than you would think, is hysterical dissociation, which is the term given to the Dr Jekyll and Mr Hyde splitting of a person's personality. In this, unknown to themselves, they live out two (or more) different identities. Whilst occupying one identity, they are incapable of recalling the other existence and quite often the two characters are poles apart. Although I have observed the phenomenon, at the time of writing I have never been consulted to assist; and since the subject is usually unaware of the existence of his own problem, I do not expect I ever will. A simpler form of this dissociation is somnambulism, where the subject walks and/or talks in his sleep but has no recall of the adventure in his normal waking state.

We have one last all-embracing 'type' to consider before we move on to the causes and cures. To explain this I have to introduce a word which is often bandied around carelessly, and which attracts a lot of different meanings in its day-to-day usage: *anxiety*.

Anxiety types

Jung described anxiety as 'fear spread thinly'; Freud talked of 'free floating anxiety, nameless, formless, and timeless, which attaches itself to nothing'. Whenever I use the word 'anxiety', I will be talking of something 'inside the person but outside his own control' – a state of anxiety (an effect) which is brought about by subconscious forces (a cause) not within the subject's intellectual awareness. We are not talking about somebody worrying over matters they are aware of, such as death, divorce, bankruptcy, etc. Nor are we talking about somebody fearing something they are aware of, such as death, divorce, bankruptcy, etc. What we are talking about is a state of anxiety from subconscious causes which is triggered off, or aggravated, by conscious associations.

Here we can be as pedantic as you like and say categorically that there cannot be an effect unless there is a cause.

CAUSE and EFFECT

Your client will willingly relate the effect (his symptoms) and quite often is only too willing to give you his interpretation of the cause (all the problems in his environment – erroneous associations, of course). It will be your job to help him discover, and/or alleviate, the true subconscious cause.

Subconscious anxiety within the human psyche is intolerable to the organism as a whole, and will produce an effect upon the organism as a whole – either mentally or physically, or a combination of both.

Reason and logic, determination and will-power, maturity and experience, persistence and patience, worry and fear – the anxious subject has used all these on his 'free floating anxiety' and it has still become remorselessly more and more intolerable. This horrifying fear of the unknown, this nameless, formless, timeless anxiety is going to find an outlet in one of three directions, as shown in Figure 1. I will explain the last one first.

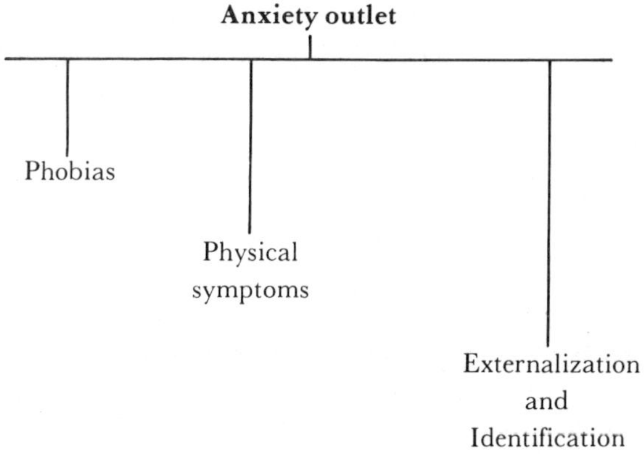

Figure 1

Externalization and Identification

The subject's subconscious anxiety is felt inwardly and projected outwardly. In effect, what is actually taking place is this:

> 'My goodness I feel anxious . . . What's the matter with me? . . . Aha!! . . . Look at that poor old lady over there with a broken leg . . . I'll go and help her! There! I feel better already.'

We are talking about a subconscious process, but the effect is very conscious. The subject worries over the worries of others, involves himself in the troubles and problems of others. As he helps them overcome their worries, troubles and problems he is symbolically dealing with his own – he is temporarily removing his own projected anxiety (until next time). Any nurse will tell you she derives a lot of personal satisfaction from her nursing. The greater the subconscious anxiety the greater the need to externalize, and most members of the healing profession are driven and motivated by such an unconscious process. Now do you realize why the suicide, divorce and alcoholism rates of psychiatrists are so high? They are at the top of the tree as anxiety subjects; they have subconsciously realized that it is a problem of the mind which they need to externalize and identify.

A word of warning and self-justification. A good therapist must be an observer but never a critic. However, he must always observe with a critical eye, and while, within this book we are offering explanations and causes of human behaviour, this should in no way be taken as a criticism. My admiration for nurses leaves me speechless, but I would still say that within six months of completing a successful psychoanalysis (of which more later) and removing her subconscious anxiety, the average nurse would resign her career! As a vocation it is first class, but as just a job of work (minus the externalization content) it just does not compute. As a point of interest, on this matter I speak from experience: I have taken more than thirty nurses through analysis and less than half are currently still nursing. I would love the opportunity to take a psychiatrist through psychoanalysis, and would hazard a good bet that he would then become a psychoanalyst, and make a very good one too.

The gain to the intellect from externalization and identification is that the unknown has been symbolically converted into the known; for, by helping and removing the troubles of others, the subject is in fact removing his own projected anxiety. This is very satisfying to the subject, and has the by-product of being extremely useful to society as a whole. But, of course, in no way does it really remove the basic subconscious anxiety that remains, like a lion in its lair, awaiting a chance and unlikely release by fate – or the more likely (and scientific) release by analysis.

Phobias

Practically every phobia you could invent (even in your wildest dreams) has been given a name. The word 'phobia' was first used to describe morbid fears by a Roman writer called Celsus almost two thousand years ago. Since him many other writers – including the great bard himself, William Shakespeare – have mentioned phobias. Most people suffer from at least one phobic fear, although it is unlikely that they have ever thought of their own particular 'silly' as being a phobia. Ladies who scuttle away when a spider appears, do not usually think of their fear as a phobia (arachnophobia), but merely as themselves being 'silly'. The man who feels almost drawn to the edge of the cliff, and who fears he might just throw himself over the edge, again only views it as himself 'being a bit stupid' – not, as it really is, a phobia (acrophobia). The person who blushes furiously if you look at him pointedly, has probably never heard of the word scopophobia (a fear of being stared at). Again, the same person, who is actually afraid of blushing, is unlikely to have heard the word ereuthophobia (fear of blushing).

Sigmund Freud knew all about hodophobia (fear of travel) – he suffered from it himself. Queen Elizabeth I knew all about anthophobia (although it is unlikely she ever heard the name) because she could not bear a rose near her. The triskaidekaphobia which beset King Edward VII caused him immense anxiety if ever there were thirteen people at a table. On one occasion he was saved from near apoplexy by the hasty explanation that one of the lady diners was pregnant; thus there were really fourteen at the table.

All phobias sound so very different: agoraphobia, meaning to be frightened of open spaces; claustrophobia, meaning to be frightened of enclosed spaces; belonophobia, a fear of sharp objects; spheksophobia, which is a fear of wasps – I know of at least two hundred I could continue listing. Yet, in my eyes, they are all the same thing: 'a symbolic outward expression of an internal anxiety'. The sufferers are all afraid of the same thing – that nameless, timeless, formless, something inside themselves, but outside their own control.

What actually happens is that the nameless, formless, timeless, free floating anxiety within the person is projected outwards (rather like externalization and identification) but attaches itself to a symbolic, real situation, or object within the environment. The symbolism varies enormously from individual to individual, but the subconscious mechanism at work is identical in all instances.

As a rule of thumb, people with very low IQs do not get

phobias because the subconscious process needs a degree of intellect to carry it to conclusion. The gain to the intellect is that the subject, instead of being frightened of something awful within himself which he cannot understand, now actually believes that he knows what he is frightened of (blood, dogs, sharp knives, etc.) and can go to the trouble of making sure that he avoids such things – effectively keeping himself free from the anxiety. Once again, the unknown has been converted to the known. There is, of course, a snag; in fact, more than one snag. The mind always hits you where it hurts you most: the opera singer will likely develop halophobia, and lose her voice; the show jumper will likely fear horses or travelling, and worse . . .

Should the subject avoid his phobic situation or object and still experience a bout of anxiety, then the process of symbolism will skilfully extend his phobia at an alarming rate. The claustrophobic, then, who started off afraid of just broom cupboards, will soon add to it an impressive list of lifts, motor cars, cinemas, theatres, buses, trams, etc., until it becomes more and more difficult to avoid each phobic situation.

Physical Symptoms

It would be a very brave man who tried to compile a list of bodily symptoms likely to be proven psychogenic. I would simply state that any physical symptom, other than injuries, may well prove to be psychosomatic or psychokinetic. The science of psychophysics has barely scratched the surface. When I say any symptom, I really do mean it. For example, Dr Richard Mackarness has written an excellent study on allergies called *Not All in the Mind* (Pan Books, 1976). With the greatest respect to the learned doctor, his book would be more aptly titled 'It's not all in the part of the mind we consciously use.' Then, I would agree with him. Ask a medical man for an explanation of an allergy, say milk, and the explanation will be stupifying: 'The enzyme action of the cholesterol fat in the amino acid reacts upon the carbohydrate protein, etc., etc.' (I hasten to add that I was there deliberately writing gibberish.) His explanation will make sense to him and he will have logically explained the rash on the skin, or whatever. Again, ask him, 'Why?' and once more he will likely go through his rigmarole of explanation. Once more, ask him 'Yes, but why?'

and you will probably be dismissed as an idiot – but really your question begs an answer. Why should one person's 'computer' go sufficiently into malfunction that it should cause the organism to reject milk? Back to our old annual 'cause and effect'. Take the person into analytical therapy (more of which later) and you would expect to make conscious a previously subconscious link between milk and anxiety. Making the anxiety 'conscious' will reveal the link to the subject's intellectual and emotional satisfaction, and the allergy will disappear. This is going to take a lot of explanation and is very hard to understand, so for now I will aim for nothing more than planting seeds. At a later time you will see how well the jigsaw is put together.

Stay within the concept of psychically created physical symptoms for a moment – and please, please, grasp that we are not talking about imaginary ailments. We are talking about symptoms as real as a hole in the stomach wall created by an action of the mind. When the stomach ulcer is healed by surgery, or medical intervention, the establishment, and indeed the subject himself, would be well content that the problem has been resolved. But you are going to realize that the anxiety which caused the effect (the symptom) is still lurking in its lair and will often repeat the process all over again. The mind carries its memory traces and patterns, and patterns are likely to be repeated. Thus, the infant that suffered through its youngest years with digestive disturbances, sickness and vomiting, has a strong memory pattern laid down, and in later years that same person will react with gastric disorder to anxiety, indeed even conscious worry and fear will go straight to his stomach.

There is a very similar gain to the intellect with bodily symptoms, as there is with phobias and with externalization – again the fear of the unknown; that nameless, formless, timeless anxiety has been replaced by the known – in this case a bodily disorder. Once again, practical remedies can be applied: just as the phobic could avoid his phobic situation so this subject can apply medicine, diet, etc., to his bodily symptoms. The tragedy, however, lies in the fact that all remedies are being applied to the effect and not the cause.

As I struggle to get points across I become increasingly aware that many of my comments will read as criticism of established medicine and the like. At the risk of being repetitive, I would like to say again that a good therapist should be an observer, without being a critic: but that nevertheless he must always observe with a critical eye. I believe that success comes only to those who are of use, and never to those who abuse, and that as a general policy we should be entirely satisfied with being right, without ever having to insist on showing that the other fellow is wrong. Freud himself said that 'there is no court to appeal to,' and that he could have wished for a bigger impact upon humanity from his writings. He realized, and philosophically accepted, something that you too must accept, otherwise you will create needless aggravation with family, friends and, indeed, clients.

As we delve deeper into human behaviour, its explanations, its causes and effects, it will not be long before we are talking very frankly on the subject of human sexuality. We would, however, be foolish if we thought others would be so frank. In the world of sexuality the subject wears 'a heavy overcoat of concealment woven of a tissue of lies'. You will come to accept – possibly you do already – that man's so-called rules for the practical regulation of sexual behaviour within society are based on hypocrisy, and display little or no common sense. What is called for by society's so-called 'morality' and the 'thou shalt not' applied to masturbation and pre-marital sex, all call for a far bigger sacrifice than they are worth and are certainly not founded on honesty. A recent well-documented investigation revealed that of 5000 women questioned between the ages of 30 and 40 years, a mind-boggling 30 per cent had never, to their knowledge, experienced a sexual orgasm. A quickly suppressed report in New Zealand, undertaken by a group of psychotherapists in the early 1970s, revealed that, of 1000 subjects investigated, *all* had been subjected to a sexual assault in their forming years and that in 35 per cent of the cases it had been carried out by a near relative. Using the words 'sexual assault' in their loosest form, I would also state categorically that I have never yet had a client successfully complete the process of analysis without he or she having recalled such a happening, and I would estimate the 35 per cent factor to be nearer 50 per cent.

Soon we will investigate the link between anxiety, fear and sexuality and you are going to have to ensure that your own prejudices (for, or against, certain subjects) do not colour and distort your own thinking on the subject. Freud was ready to admit that his own researches and investigations occasionally found an internal resistance 'presumably from the depths of his own neuroses', and you too must be open-minded enough to admit to a similar possibility within yourself.

ANXIETY – the actual 'anxiety attack'

Whenever dealing with an anxiety subject, who stutters or stammers, has a nervous twitch, has a phobia or bodily symptom, or who suffers depression or any of the faulty behaviour patterns already mentioned, you will come across an experience known as the anxiety attack.

The phobic would almost certainly experience it, or part of it, when confronted with his phobic situation or object. But before I describe the attack in full, please understand that it is a progressive situation, and that many subjects would experience only the first part, and so the latter part of the description would mean nothing to them. I advocate learning the description of the anxiety attack parrot fashion, word perfect, so that you can ask your client whether he has ever experienced such a phenomenon. This will serve a twofold purpose: one, it will give you an indication of the severity of the problem, and two, it will impress, and therefore reassure, your client as to the depth of your insight into his problem. Plenty of people will say, 'Yes, that's it exactly.'

The attack usually comes with little or no warning and for no apparent cause or reason that the subject can satisfactorily explain to himself. It is truly the fear of the unknown.

> The heart beats alarmingly quickly – like a palpitation, and the subject becomes vaguely aware of a number of bodily effects. Frequently the breathing rate increases as rapidly as though the subject just wasn't getting enough air. This is known as 'air hunger'. There can be a cramped feeling across the lower part of the diaphragm and a tingling sensation, accompanied by either a hot or cold flush in unexpected parts of the body, usually the extremities – finger ends and the like. All the feelings combine to somehow vaguely suggest to the subject the advent of unconsciousness, and the person can appear almost rooted to the spot as though he had seen an apparition. He is usually struck dumb

> and immobilized, and he can neither run nor fight because it all comes from within. He is panic-struck by what is taking place, yet something, very vague, and very abstract, does present itself to him – only he cannot understand it. It is truly the unknown.

The anxiety attack was what Freud had in mind when he wrote of 'free floating anxiety', meaning that it was free of any known cause and just literally floated within the mind.

The aftermath of the anxiety attack is a return to normal, and on the surface little or no harm has been done. The subject has certainly received an unpleasant experience; he can neither explain it to his own satisfaction, nor yet can he begin to understand it. One thing it has done is to lay down a very strong memory pattern, or trace; and herein lies the true size of the iceberg of which we have only observed the tip. One school of psychology likens it to living alongside a volcano which appears quiet, but which without you knowing in advance, may erupt at any moment.

The victim of the anxiety attack begins to feel like that about his own being – he's watching and waiting for the next eruption and by so doing possibly ensuring the arrival of the attack. What we know for definite is that the memory trace, the pattern, will be closely followed at second or subsequent attacks, and just like that volcano will cut deeper and deeper furrows and spread further and further in area.

In the anxiety attack there is a classic example of mind reacting upon body, and of body reacting upon mind; the whole thing gathering force and momentum until a discharge takes place and the pent-up energy dissipates. I promise you my motives are not crude or vulgar when I ask you for a moment to consider another aspect of human behaviour where that occurs – namely, sexuality. Here mind reacts upon body, body reacts upon mind, and the whole thing gathers force and momentum until a discharge takes place and the pent-up energy dissipates. We are still doing a jigsaw, but you will see that all the pieces fit neatly together to make a picture in due course, and that the comparison of the anxiety attack with sexual intercourse is no idle choice of words.

At the moment we are still working a little upside-down. We have looked at completed sections of our jigsaw, out of which we eventually aim to make a picture, but have yet to look at how those completed sections are created. Look again at those, so recognizable, character types; and now let's step back in time, to see what causes produced those effects. Oh yes, we still abide by our principal rule that you cannot have an effect without a cause. Now we say the effect is a certain type of character, so we will go searching for causes of that effect.

On our search for enlightenment we will need to be as inquisitive for information as would be a learning infant, but one whose enquiries go way beyond, for example, why a round ball rolls and a square cube doesn't, and whose researches cause him to question the mystery of life itself, how babies are made, the difference between the sexes and so forth. Let us in our turn start with one of the mysteries – putting aside any personal opinions about the controversy between Darwin's exposition of evolution and Genesis or biblical accounts of creation, and simply confine ourselves to provables.

As a physical organism we are inherently bisexual. Examine either sex and you will find attributes of the other sex within the blood, the cells and the genitals. These are distinct things which no man of reason could deny, part of the mammary glands evident on the male; an atrophied penis (the clitoris) evident on the female, and so on. We make a firm platform on which to begin if we stick with the opening sentence that as a physical organism we are inherently bisexual, and that such opposite sexual characteristics are born in us, and have so been since time immemorial. That such a conclusion adds more weight to Darwin's explanation that we come originally from a single sex species does not concern us at this point; our researches have other paths to follow.

The rate at which our species is proliferating over the planet is abundant evidence of the fact that this physical bisexuality is carried forward into psychical reality in only a minority of cases; and the obvious selfishness of our genes infers that those who defy the duty of procreation imposed on them by the subconscious instinct of self-preservation which governs us all, must inevitably be construed as being in the grip of a behavioural disorder every bit as explainable as claustrophobia. Forgive me if I hurry on, having planted only a tiny seed, as the controversial subject of homosexuality and the like is too big a bone to chew on – yet – I can already hear one or two of you saying that you had no intention, or wish, to look as deeply into the human psyche as it now becomes obvious that we are doing; that perhaps you just wanted to learn how to hypnotize people and so help them. Let me say now that if you really do feel like that, you should put the book down now; for soon you will reach what a pilot calls 'vee one', where he has to take off, whether he wants to or not. You in your turn will find that your understanding of human character formation will almost certainly light a fire of consuming curiosity within you that may well channel much of your future life for you.

It had been my intention when I started writing this book to sacrifice some of my own beliefs and awareness at the altar of expediency, but I have decided that I will not, indeed cannot. A true understanding of what I impart will bring you to the use of a word which very few hypnotherapists or psychotherapists use, the word 'cure'. Most therapists would say that at best they aimed to help people, and many disciplines would expressly forbid the use of the word at all, other than in the negative form. A doctor would presumably claim a cure for migraine, for example, if the pains responded to his pills or potion, but would the title really be deserved if the migraines returned – however well they again responded to the treatment? Would it not be fairer, and more honest, to claim a cure only if the migraines went, never to return, and with no recourse to dietary or environmental control?

This use of the word 'cure' is going to strike to the very roots of our subject. Remember I said hypnosis alone achieved nothing, but was akin to the surgeon's scalpel. Well, now let me rephrase something, and say that hypnosis can be used to aid the power of suggestion which will attempt a control of a problem; or hypnosis can be used as an aid to recall, to assist a process called psychoanalysis, designed to find, and remove, originating causes of people's behavioural disorders, and, in the process of removal, to cure the problem. Bring it down to its simplest explainable form and think of the plump subject seeking the help of the therapist to lose some weight.

Method 1: Use the hypnotic state to aid the power of suggestion and give post-hypnotic suggestion and aversion therapy designed to help the person control his eating pattern. The subject would normally be agreeably surprised at how easy the whole thing became – for the next few weeks – and would remain your staunchest advocate even if he subsequently put all the weight back on.

Method 2: Stand firmly by the doctrine of cause and effect. Look at the eating as a 'compulsive activity' inside the person but outside their own control. Use the hypnotic state as an aid to recall, to find and remove the true originating causes of the subject's desire for 'oral satisfaction' and cure the problem so that the person has no further need for dietary control – eating only when hungry as opposed to compulsion.

Unfortunately method 2 is far more troublesome to both client and therapist and will take a number of sessions. The client will strongly doubt both the necessity for, and potential efficacy of, such a method. Since the client has no conception of 'what they could be like', if they 'were not as they are', most clients would likely opt for method 1. I would content myself with explaining the difference between suggestion and analytical therapy, in so far as such a thing is explainable in lay terms, stressing the difference between control and cure.

I previously mentioned I would content myself with knowing I was right, without having to prove the client wrong. Should the client prefer to believe that his 'compulsive activity' – his compulsive eating – is brought about by greed, a sweet tooth and conscious worries – well, it's his mind and his own body.

Experience proves that many clients who have a single session of suggestion therapy for weight control return months later, quite often ready, and prepared for, method 2.

3.
Character Formation

EARLY DEVELOPMENT – The forming years

Most, but of course not all, schools or disciplines of psychology are agreed upon the pressures on us, and our reaction to those pressures, which exist through our forming years. It is only the threat of possible retribution which forces me to couch it all in my own words rather than reprinting exactly from other writings. Remember we said there was the oral period of development, the anal period and the genital stage. We will take them one at a time, bearing in mind that we are talking of 'the norm' and not 'institutionalized upbringings'.

Our love at first is narcissistic and, at that very, very early stage of our lives, being aware only of ourselves, we have only ourselves to blame if things go wrong. We soon become aware of the existence of another important being in our lives, our mother. We give her our love unquestioningly because she brings those three vital and important requirements we will treasure all our lives: *love, nourishment* and *security*. These three things, albeit given different names, we will want for the rest of our lives. We will each react in our own particular way if we lose any one, or all three, and it is the way we learn to react in our earliest years which predisposes us to react in exactly the same way for the rest of our lives.

Unquestionably the two strongest instinctual forces which drive us are:

1. the instinct of self preservation;
2. the instinct of procreation.

Follow Darwin's route back far enough and we would have to believe that the mouth was once a sexual orifice. Be that as it may, it certainly is the focal point of a baby's pleasure drive, and the action of sucking, which very naturally satisfies the instinct of self-preservation, also brings a mixture of anticipation, excitement, and self-gratification, and quite understandably the infant resents any interference that takes place. However, doorbells do ring, pans boil over, TV channels need changing and though the infant has no awareness of these things, there are nevertheless interruptions to our hero's pleasure and self-gratification. Here then comes our first frustration in life, but being narcissistic still, we feel this frustration as a self-frustration, and rage and resentment can be promptly turned inwards to the self.

Many adults carry this predisposition and have inward tempers and rages. Armed with maturity, though, the adult does not turn that inward rage against himself, but points it outwards and with careless aim at the 'guilty' part of the environment. Not so the infant, still too undeveloped actually to understand these frustrations and rages; they are simply directed towards ourselves and lead to self-condemnation and self-disparagement and an overwhelming feeling of depression. This inward raging can become a predisposition which in later life will cause depression, melancholia or agitated melancholia. Naturally our rage could be outward and very evident, and that would predispose us to be able to get rid of our pent-up emotions in later life.

We don't have to rage at the interruption of our pleasures. We could be far more apathetic and just withdraw. Give up the pleasure, dissociate one from the other. Dissociate the pleasure from the activity, so the activity just becomes a bore, a stereotyped thing devoid of pleasure, while the pleasure, which is actually the very embryo of our feelings, and even sexual urges, is pushed firmly under, so lying dormant and unused. It will emerge eventually but when it does it will be in a form and shape scarcely recognizable as that original, intensely pleasurable bodily instinct.

As we continue the explanation of the earliest feelings, do not allow any thoughts of reasoning ability to cloud the issues. As infants we are still incapable of reasoning, as yet only concerned with what is happening or what has happened and have no conception of what is likely to happen. Feelings are absolute, 'all or nothing', bright and elated or abysmally depressed. We have many things to experience before we realize it does not have to be 'all or nothing', that in fact there are an infinite number of points on the compass between.

Whether boy or girl, we are still only aware of our father in the background – vague and shadowy, dim and impersonal. But the developing mind is becoming something else, not just an infant any more, but a boy infant or a girl infant – as the case may be.

The Girl Child

In the backs of our minds let us keep the thought that a girl's very first love ever was for a person of the same sex. The sexual content of our loving is of course not yet discernible; indeed, if you apply adult standards; it is not even present. But we are not applying adult standards, we are talking about a mind which absorbs without criticism. For the girl, with the advent of her femininity comes the first inner conflict to face and fight out. That dim, impersonal figure in the background is going to prove to be a man. As human as Mother, but different and somehow dangerous and exciting. Somehow to that young mind it is all a threat, complications that strike at that love, nourishment and security arrangement, that exists with Mother; for the father is a man, and he is Mother's, and if one loves him too then it might mean losing the love of Mother. And yet our girl heroine cannot help herself, her dawning sexuality and femininity drive her, and she does aspire to Father's love. It fascinates her. The first true conflict within her psyche has arisen, but this conflict is probably the biggest subconscious conflict she will ever face. The conflict is no less than a collision between our two greatest instinctual drives: the instinct of self-preservation, or rather Mother, with the love, nourishment and security; versus the instinct of procreation, or rather Father, the man, with the consequent danger and excitement. In a normal development stream our girl heroine never, in fact, has to make such a momentous choice: all she does is worry about it as though she had to. The anxiety takes place at a subconscious level, the worry takes place outwardly. All these powerful interacting forces are part of natural development in our earliest months and do not, of necessity, have to have bad effects upon us later. Should we experience an undisturbed and amiably loving relationship with Mother, where we feel loved and needed, then our feelings will develop naturally. If we feel secure then we will not be predisposed towards inferiority and will be well equipped for all the other momentous decisions of later life.

The Boy Child

Whether boy or girl we will still face conflict in those early months, and a boy's development and conflict is along similar lines to the girl's.

Again the dawning of sexuality, the beginning of masculinity, when the infant starts to become a boy infant, is the advent of conflict. Our boy hero sees that Mother is a woman and also sees that Father is a man. I say 'sees', rather than 'realizes', because no reasoning is applied at all. The feelings come from within. What the boy finds is feelings within himself. He experiences rivalry. Father is a rival for the love of Mother, and Mother represents security at grass roots. Mother brings love, nourishment and security, and even in the earliest years and months his loving has an erotic content (again not when judged by adult standards though). Other feelings emerge: hate, jealousy, and guilt. The boy child is confused. Again it is the momentous clash between those two main instinctual drives: self-preservation to which Father is very obviously a threat, as far as our hero is concerned, and procreation, symbolized by Mother. The struggle going on inside his mind is totally subconscious and is demonstrated outwardly in ordinary worry. Again these complex forces do not necessarily lead to compensatory behaviour in later life. Every last one of us, experiencing a normal development stream, takes a bite from these cherries, and only where the bite is too large or too little does it lead to malfunction.

Perception

As the months go by in this oral period of development other chances of conflict occur.

There are other people beside Mother and Father, and other events beside feeding and self-gratification. We learn that if you fall or bang your head it hurts, and that if you cut yourself you bleed. These events, these things, these beings, have a nasty habit of reacting in their own way, and not necessarily in a nice way. The growing mind is beginning to reason, beginning to realize, that there is more than just what has happened, more than just what is happening, there is also what might happen. So other feelings are being born and used. We imagine what might happen, we anticipate what might happen, we can be apprehensive about what might happen, we can be jealous about what might happen, and we can be suspicious of what might happen. We are becoming predisposed to react in a certain way to events in our life. Of course, as Epictetus wrote so clearly in 3000 BC, 'Men are not the least influenced by events, but only by their interpretation of those events', so the predisposition varies as infinitely as does the interpretation – from individual to individual.

In those early months the infant will find that in order to survive he will need to seek the pleasure of feeding. At this stage it would be fair to say the whole of the sexual instinct is turned inwards and all the pleasurable bodily instincts are in the mouth. The more we suck, the more pleasure we get, the more likely we are to survive. The two basic instincts are reacting upon each other. Take away the bottle, or the breast, and the infant will react as previously described. Because the action is so pleasurable, the infant may try some more learning of its own, and learn how to create such a pleasure for itself, by imitating that action of feeding – but minus the presence of a teat or nipple. The mouth is opened and the tongue pushed vigorously back and forth, to bring pleasure and satisfaction to the organism. There, we have learned self-gratification – what is termed 'oral satisfaction'. This particular predisposition may well play an important part in our lives, leading to a predisposition towards oral satisfaction in its many and varied forms. Thumb-sucking, nail-biting, compulsive eating, smoking, gum-chewing, lip-chewing, to name but a few – to say little of the amount of oral activity taken forward in the development of the sexuality of the individual.

All these feelings which we gather and gain by experience as we go along are determining bit by bit the way in which we will behave in future. Assume the infant was to be, or felt itself to be, deprived in some way; let's say of mother love. Be assured that throughout his entire life he will carry a feeling of deprivation that will tinge everything he does. These subtle, confused and often immensely complex feelings of oral days are carried forward to maturity.

Try to define predisposition away from the dictionary and we talk of a trend, a tendency to react to new events and situations in the environment in the way in which we reacted to the old events and situations in the environment. All human behaviour is learned, and the behaviourists, amongst modern therapies, would have us believe, that what has been learned can be unlearned. Whereas this doctrine is in essence correct, we who are to adopt the doctrine of cause and effect are going to realize that it is no good teaching an old dog new tricks – if, amid that range of new tricks, he also starts to mess the carpet. Small compensation to the agoraphobic to be taught how to control and overcome his agoraphobia, if the subconscious causes find their outlet in an alternative, far more punishing, and far more restrictive way, than ever the fear of open spaces had been. One thing we can be sure of is that where a subconscious conflict is at work producing a symptom, be it any one of our three types of symptom (bodily symptom, phobia, or externalization and identification) then the mind will always hit where it hurts most. The opera singer loses the voice, the mathematician gets a constant head pain, and so on; and to say again, small compensation to the phobic person to be helped to overcome his phobia, only to find he is covered from head to foot in a nervous rash or whatever.

We have looked at some of the many complex factors which can help to produce an 'oral type' of personality in later life. Deep in themselves oral folk tend to be rather insecure and very easily hurt. Indeed, this predisposition to react inwardly to criticism creates a compensation which, like the double-edged sword it is, cuts deeper into them. Because they are hurt so easily themselves they overcompensate to avoid hurting others. Indeed, if they do hurt others, it tends to hurt them more! Because of this they are easy meat to the bully and tyrant. One of the inherent tragedies of human behaviour is that the soft and gentle oral type with his day-dreaming ways is often attracted to the bluster and power of the 'anal' type who makes his life an absolute misery. With his intuitive understanding, our oral type eventually sees through the anal type's paranoid ways to the shallowness underneath, but by then it is often too late – wedding bells have rung or a relationship has become established. There is really only one hope for our oral type, one possibility of true expression (because he feels everything inwardly his feelings have an intensity unparalleled by any of the other character types). It is an inward thing, so he finds it difficult to express these feelings outwardly. However, all that feeling working away inside has immense possibilities of creation. Should our oral type only discover the outlet for that creativity – be it art, music, writing or whatever – then he has found the one true means of outward expression.

Anal Development

Usually about the age of $2\frac{1}{2}$ – 3 years our boy and girl infants start to enter the second development phase – they cease to be 'babies' and become infants and toddlers, and are no longer helpless and totally dependent beings. They are finding out that if they want something there are ways of getting it. Their demands and entreaties can produce effects. More and more they become aware of the environment: round balls roll along the carpet, square cubes have to be pushed, hot things burn, cold things freeze, sharp things cut, fragile things break, knocks, bangs and falls hurt. This time is called the anal period for good reason, for just as the intensity of oral experience lent its name to the development period, now our hero is coerced to make that momentous step – bowel control.

A lot of attention is paid to this aspect by others: should he do as 'they' want him to, he is praised and rewarded; should he fail or defy 'them', there can be punishment – if only the taking away of those basic requirements he has learnt to look forward to so much: love, nourishment and security. Accidents do happen, and he, who views his faeces as just a part of himself, is baffled and bemused by these imponderable influences being brought to bear upon him. As a perfect demonstration of the love he feels, he will reach into a soiled nappy and eagerly hold out in both hands a part of himself as a gift to the one he loves. The displeasure and subsequent washing is as puzzling as the rejection of his sacrifice.

All this time he is learning, and learning to exert his own will on others. He can demand things as of his right, he can plead for things, and even learn to deceive by pretending. With biting teeth and pinching fingers he learns to inflict suffering upon others, and he is totally reckless as to the consequences. He neither sees, nor cares, about the extent of the suffering he causes, not as yet having developed any feeling for the needs or problems of others. He can be dreadfully sadistic with his play, which is why some disciplines of psychology refer to this as the anal/sadistic period.

The passing of faeces may be pleasurable, and the embryo of anal eroticism is born. Should he feel guilty about this pleasure, the eroticism will likely be inverted to an intense distaste. More and more you will see the dextrous way in which the human mind will completely invert something, or even invert and project outwards. Listen to the bravado of a youth about to go out and 'bash some queers' because he 'hates all queers', and be confident that same youth is probably latently homosexual, and would really like to 'bash' the feelings out of himself. Always suspect a subconscious opposite if 'Young Cassius doth protest too much his innocence for to proclaim'.

Genital Development

And so, into the genital period of development, and the pleasures of what is termed pre-puberty masturbation, although the title 'masturbation' is scarcely warranted, consisting as it does of an inquisitive fiddling and an awareness of pleasurable sensation. This precursor of sexual arousal, merely a sensual tingle, can be experienced on a swing, when lifted up quickly, on a slide, by squeezing the knees together in the bath, and so on. Our hero will find some methods for sure, and just as likely heap a whole load of controversy upon his young shoulders: 'Leave it alone, the birds will think it's a worm'; 'Don't fiddle with it, the ducks will get it'; 'Sit with your knees together, little girl' and so on.

Soon, the startled gaze of that young child has to observe another amazing phenomenon: we are not all the same. Little boys have a 'willy' and little girls don't. Surprise! Surprise! Now, you get all sorts of different reactions. Some little boys will make their assumption in a flash (pardon the pun). 'Well,' they say, 'what a pathetic creature the girl is – hasn't even got one – useless creatures'. There is your 'male chauvinist pig' of later life, who thinks that all women are useless. Tell him where his original opinion came from, and he'll laugh at you in disbelief.

Some little girls, not realizing that it's all little girls, and not just them, feel distinctly inferior, or even jealous. It's as though he got something for Christmas she didn't. It may even cause her to make a very critical examination of herself, sometimes even with the aid of a mirror. Sometimes she will find one (remember the clitoris is, biologically speaking, an atrophied penis) but the size of it does little for her ego development.

The thousands of different reactions to this puzzling phenomenon vary from total disinterest, or even disavowal (a flat refusal to believe what they have seen) to, at the other extreme, a horror that they themselves must be deformed. None of it, however, does anything to dampen the ever-growing curiosity of that ever-expanding mind which is still gathering information and learning behaviour – until, that is, it has learned sufficient to carry out its appointed task – the procreation of the species, which from puberty on will be capable of, but not necessarily willing to do.

There is another, perhaps even bigger, mystery for that young mind to ratify in this genital period of development. The mystery is to do with blood. Can it be true, says that young enquiring mind, that girls actually bleed from 'down there'? That can't be true, surely? You only get blood if you cut yourself – that has been painfully discovered already – and yet – sometimes there is the evidence of one's own eyes to convince one – perhaps the sight of blood down the toilet, or the discovery of a used sanitary towel – the graphic and elaborate description provided by an elder brother or sister – or the well-meaning instruction of an adult – and yet – it scarcely seems believable – blood from 'there'!

Well, I have an explanation. Now my explanation is stupid, and I know it, but, there again, I am not a five-year-old. My explanation is this: Suppose, just suppose, that all little girls and all little boys were born exactly the same – and – for some reason, little girls had 'theirs' *cut off.* Now, if that doesn't explain the *blood*, and if that doesn't explain the *difference*, I don't know what does. And, it's not all that difficult to figure out who would do it; because dentists will pull your teeth out and leave a gaping hole gushing blood, and doctors will cut you open and take out your appendix or tonsils, and Mum and Dad can be very cross – and they do say some funny things, these grown-ups: 'Leave it alone, the birds will think it's a worm'; 'Put it away or the ducks will bite it off'; 'Wet the bed once more and you'll get it cut off'. Suppose, just suppose, 'they' really meant it. Suppose the ultimate penalty for naughtiness was a sharp knife or a sharp pair of scissors and . . .

I did say my explanation was silly, didn't I, and of course, so it is. But for all that, at a totally subconscious level, these impressions and fantasies of youth can produce an anxiety about the possibility (if you are a boy) or the acceptance (if you are a girl), of castration.

The ever-enquiring, growing mind gets its answers, of course, and a full understanding naturally follows. In the girl's case that understanding arrives somewhat earlier than the boy's (usually) as the 'inevitability of fate' catches up with her – when she menstruates for the very first time. At school it tended to fall into two camps – those who had started, and those who hadn't. One day she was a 'had not', the next day a 'had'. Quite frequently she had thought she was looking forward to getting it over and done with, but sometimes she can find herself in the grip of an emotion she just cannot explain to herself. As childhood flies out of the window, as she gathers up the 'yoke' of her womanhood, as she receives that prison sentence of 'the curse', each month, every month for the next three of four decades, she can find herself experiencing an emotion as strong as if someone close had died – as if something was lost, and lost forever, as indeed childhood really is.

One more natural psychological gate to open. Soon the organism will be ready to carry out that requirement of the species, its appointed task of procreation. That psychological gate is: the very first ejaculation/orgasm, quite frequently accompanied by a shocked – surprised – disbelief – puzzlement – disgust – again the reaction varies enormously.

Well, we've done it, give or take a few thousand experiences. We have made it to puberty, to the magical teens, and time to start putting all that learning into practice. Our characters are well and truly formed and our predispositions well and truly established.

Repeating the philosopher Epictetus: 'Men are not . . . influenced by events, but only by their interpretation of those events' and, thanks to the uniqueness of our ability to interpret, we are all, thank goodness, going to be uniquely different from each other – but only within the bounds of certain broad guidelines: we are, after all, only human.

4.
ANXIETY AND SEXUALITY

Your understanding of what now follows is absolutely vital to your future understanding of these writings, and even more vital to your insight into human behaviour, and your future ability as a therapist – and please, I am still asking you to read this book as though you intend to become one.

I propose to explain how a cross-over can occur to our two greatest biological instincts – the instinct of self-preservation, and the instinct of procreation. Firstly, you have to grasp the correlation between fear and sexuality, and the two, at first, seem unlikely bedfellows.

FEAR and SEXUALITY – a link

Fear: a painful emotion aroused by a sense of impending danger.

In the presence of danger the whole organism is poised and alerted – poised to fight ... or ... flight. The heart beats faster and the adrenalin flows. This is no time to be day-dreaming about sexuality – that is pruned right back, as all the defence and offence mechanisms of the body are put on full alert.

Fine – now step back in time a few million years, back down that evolutionary path. That is fairly easy to do by observing the behaviour of other herding, gregarious animals like ourselves (as we were), only on the lower rungs of the evolutionary ladder. Watch a herd of buffalo, bison, wild-beast, etc. and watch the males competing for the females – quite often extremely aggressively. Obviously it makes sound biological sense that the species – which wishes to survive – should be propagated, by a process of natural selection, by the fittest, healthiest and most virile and aggressive of their number. That way the continuity of the species is more likely. So what happens? There is a fight and to the victor go the spoils. In other words the instinct of self-preservation has been used, and then followed by the instinct of procreation. There was a threat, there was a danger, there was a feedback of mastery when the danger was overcome, and then there was sexuality. We have even observed that there is an element of aggression in the make-up of sexuality.

Man, of all the animals, is the one most given to reason and logic. But still, within what Jung called 'the old mind' – if you like, the subconscious – are instincts and traces of our forefathers.

And what proof do we have?

Consult the birth statistics of a nation after time of war – sky high! Ask any man who has been 'over the top' with machine gun blazing. Ask him what he felt when he reached the safety of a dug-out – amazed at an arousal! Ask a fighter pilot what he felt like when he landed safely after aerial combat – ditto! At the lowest end of the scale, ask the young girl whether she said 'Yes' before, or after, a high-speed dash on a powerful motorbike, when she felt so afraid and exhilarated.

The aftermath of danger – once the danger has been met and overcome – is a return to normal, and then an arousal of the sexual factor. Nature has very neatly made sure, as far as possible, that the species will survive by building in a mechanism which ensures that, after a situation is confronted where a species could be decimated, then the losses are likely to be repleted by 'appropriate action' – an upsurge of sexuality. It matters not whether the fear has been logically thought out, or even recognized. This is clearly demonstrated by the lower animal orders, who still make use of this function without having the reasoning capacity to interpret their fear correctly.

Once you have grasped the basic link that fear first inhibits and then secondly arouses our sexuality, we can move on.

Remember, Jung said anxiety was 'fear spread thinly', and we have decided that a state of anxiety comes from within the psyche (that perennial something, inside the person but outside his own control). Are you ahead of me yet? The person feels anxious (fear spread thinly). He is afraid of something nameless, formless and timeless within himself. What does that do to his sexuality? You guessed! It inhibits it. Fear inhibits sexuality, and of course anxiety does the same.

Ah! But from where do such people get their feedback of mastery at overcoming danger, so that their sexuality can be restored to normal, and then raised? You guessed again! *They don't.*

So – now we can make a pedantic statement. The anxious person has an inhibition in his sexual factor, whether he knows it or not.

Now, your claustrophobic will willingly present you the symptoms of his claustrophobia, but not so his sexuality – there he will wear that heavy overcoat of concealment. Should you tell him his sexuality and his phobia are interrelated, you will likely be branded 'Crank – psychotherapists are all the same, think sex is at the root of everything', and your client will go off to a more 'understanding' therapist. You do not need to tell him anyway. You can content yourself with knowing that you are right, and waiting for him to get the same insight through your ministrations. He will realize then, that we do not think that sex is the root cause of everything. Instead we think that it is not possible to view the two things – sexuality and phobia – as separate. You cannot have one set of standards for other aspects of your life, and an entirely separate set of standards and guidelines for your sexuality. In order to discuss life, to discuss a person's problems, it is not possible to exclude his sexuality.

A point of clarification: we have said that the sexuality of an anxiety subject is inhibited. We have not said that it is non-existent. Our client may proudly claim to function sexually five times nightly, and he won't see what is plain to us – that he is emotionally anaesthetized. An inhibition in the sexual factor can be as slight as a need to 'bite' at the moment of ejaculation, or as total as psychical impotence – fetishes, sadism, masochism, transvestism, bisexuality, homosexuality. They are all 'inhibitions of the sexual factor', to a greater or lesser degree.

A few times I have mentioned the almost uncanny way in which things can be transposed in the human mind. Hate is akin to love, or put another way, 'You cannot hate, till first you have felt love.' The message is clear. The mind will happily turn something upside-down.

Many times in therapy I will deduce (inwardly) from my early questioning of a lady client, that she was one of that apparent 30 per cent who never climaxed, merely because of the symptoms she was enumerating. Of course she never mentions that as a symptom; and, unless the problems she consulted with were obviously sexual, neither would I. At a later time when she confided that it was a problem to her because she climaxed prematurely, I would not view my original inward deduction as 'wrong' – merely 'upside-down'. Perversions are reversals – turnings upside-down by the mind.

I hope you have clearly seen the link between fear and sexuality, because I now want you to be able to look at that upside-down:

The existence of ANXIETY represses or inhibits SEXUALITY.

Inhibited or repressed SEXUALITY produces ANXIETY.

I hope that having had to turn the page upside-down to read it will have branded it deeply within your mind (the meaning, not the anxiety).

Let's take a very simple and extremely basic example. Eneurisis (bedwetting): Imagine a young lad being made to feel guilty about this, and let us assume the guilt was strong enough to penetrate the subconscious (let it pass as briefly as that for now, since we will be talking about the subconscious, in depth, later). So now we have guilt at subconscious level over urinal discharge. Would you be surprised to find that the same lad felt subconsciously guilty, at a later time, over another type of discharge – an ejaculation? (Urinating, from a purely psychological point of view, is in fact a base form of ejaculation, the former being the precursor of the latter. In the younger years there is as much sensuality of feeling attached to urinating as there is sexuality attached later to ejaculation). Our poor confused lad who felt subconsciously guilty over the ejaculation has met all our requirements to produce anxiety. His sexuality is inhibited or repressed and this brings the existence of anxiety. But, because it is subconscious, he doesn't know what is causing the anxiety. The more anxiety he feels, the more his sexuality is inhibited. Boy! Has that wheel started rolling now. He has to rationalize the anxiety – or go crazy; so he disposes of the anxiety in one of three ways, shown in Figure 2.

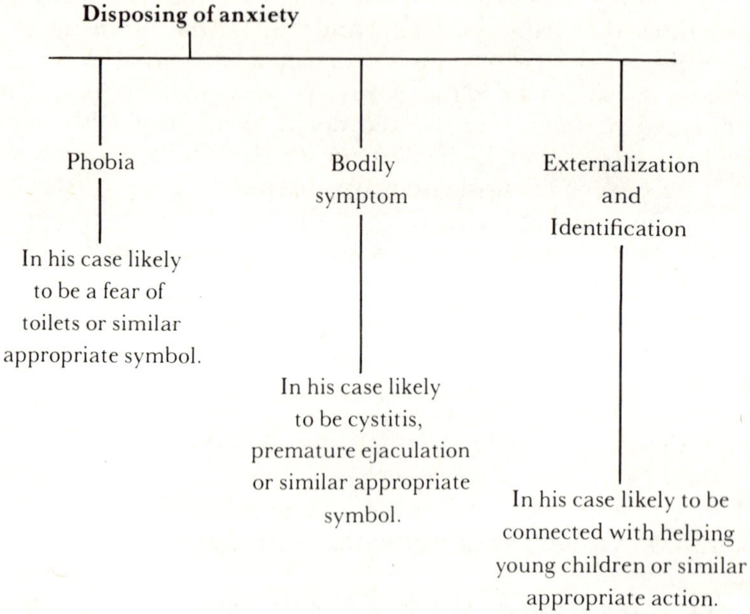

Figure 2

The conversion of sexual energy into anxiety has been cited as Nature's most severe and damaging retribution. The process of fear becoming sexually stimulating is a perfectly normal, but seldom realized, example of the same process upside-down, or reversed.

DECIDING ANALYSIS OR SUGGESTION

Earlier we said that suggestion therapy acted upon the symptoms and that analytical therapy acted upon the causes, and I would stand by that. However, to be completely fair to suggestion therapy, one has to concede that when it is applied during a hypnosis session the suggestions are inevitably having an effect upon the cause as well, in as much as the suggestions for 'calmness' and 'relaxation' react, at a subconscious level, on the subconscious anxiety.

Now a question of degree enters into the calculations. Using a most basic and perhaps trivial example, consider three cigarette smokers. We stand by the doctrine of cause and effect, and maintain that the smoking is really a 'compulsive activity' designed to create 'oral satisfaction'.

(A) One smokes 20 a day, is free from phobias, appears psychologically stable, and generally free from major inhibitions.
(B) Another one smokes 40 a day, has a phobia of spiders and heights, appears psychologically stable, and generally free from major inhibitions although is obviously prone to easy blushing.
(C) The third one smokes 70 a day, and has a peculiar mannerism which accompanies each drag on the cigarette, has phobias about snakes, rats, worms, blood and sharp knives, and, although apparently psychologically stable, has a 'hand-washing' mannerism which accompanies his talking and generally has a brooding and rather narrow-minded sort of outlook.

Fairly obviously the first one (A) will likely respond to suggestion therapy to stop smoking. The suggestions can be worded also to counter any likely alternative, such as nail-biting or compulsive eating. The general pacifying effect on the central nervous system of the hypnotic experience should combine to counter the inner anxiety for a while – certainly sufficient time for the smoking activity to cease. This will likely produce a client who believes 'it' worked for him and who is agreeably surprised at the ease with which he stops. All in all he's happy, you're happy, and he will likely recommend you everywhere he goes.

The second one (B) is far less likely to be able to respond to suggestion therapy. The therapist cannot cast doubt by inferring that 'it' might not work, so should content himself with explaining the difference between suggestion and analytical therapy. He should point out that what he is going to proceed with aims at 'control' as opposed to 'cure' and that perhaps some time the client might like to return to have subconscious causes removed. Should the smoker then find, after a few days, that the inner anxiety was so strong he was compelled to resume his compulsive activity (start smoking again) then he may well return for treatment. At that stage it would be almost false pretences to repeat suggestion therapy, because if he couldn't respond to 'it' the first time, he is even less likely to be able to the second.

What about (C)? If you have not recognized our old friend the obsessional, then you should have done. This person doesn't usually present himself for therapy. He could stop smoking any time that he wanted to. No hypnotist could ever 'conquer his mind', etc., etc. Should he come for treatment then he probably has a subconscious reason. He'd love to be able to tell them all in the pub how 'his mind was too strong' for that hypnotist chap (he'd be puffing contentedly on his cigarette, mind you, at the time). His smoking is not compulsive – it is an obsession, and if he goes to an acupuncturist, he will likely be given a tiny wire in the ear he can fiddle with from time to time. I would be the first to give him the address of the nearest acupuncturist. Under no circumstances would I ever attempt suggestion therapy; and I should think hard and long before I took him into analytical therapy. Even if I did, I would estimate my chances of success as some 80 per cent lower than 'the norm' – and I would tell him so. In analytical therapy the introduction of a doubt is not so relevant as suggestion therapy, and since the person is spending money he has got a right to know the truth. One good thing about our obsessional: he knows he's obsessional all right. He'll even put it forward spontaneously and so there is no fear of insulting him.

So you see, the severity of symptoms is going to play a part in the manner in which we shall learn to deal with them; and to that there is another imponderable – we are seeing the symptoms as they are now, in accordance with pressures of the environment as they are now. Look at the same symptoms again six months later when the client has won the football pools, and you will likely see them recede. Look again six months later when he has gone bankrupt, and you will likely see them back again – tenfold.

THE OEDIPUS COMPLEX

Man, of all the animals on the face of the earth, is the one predisposed to neuroses. Take any animal away from its natural environment, educate it away from its instincts, and you run the risk of a neurosis – crib-biting in stabled horses, head-swaying in caged lions; there are many examples within the animal world. Man, however, has the dubious distinction of being the only one predisposed to neurotic behaviour, being educated almost completely away from his instincts.

Step a rung down that evolutionary ladder again, and look at man demonstrating the herding gregariousness of his species as wandering bands of nomads, complete with herd leader and territorial rights. (Are we so very different today, I wonder, with our housing estates and political leaders?) Ask yourself, 'Who would have mated with whom?' Would the 'tribe' have waited for a chance and unlikely encounter with another wandering tribe; or is it more likely that mating would have taken place between tribe members, with the 'herd leader' taking first choice? What I am trying to say, as tactfully as possible, is that man's sexual instinct is, at its grass roots, incestuous, and that particular bit of 'naughtiness' has to be educated out of his playtime at a very early age.

Far be it from me to advocate incestuous relationships as the latest 'in' therapy for neurosis. I aim merely to explain the effect upon the psyche of being turned away from it – and this particular bit of education is usually complete by about age seven or so. Ask any mother at what age our boy hero became capable of an erection and she will confirm that it was literally from the earliest hours of his life, and that at bathtime, and nappy-changing times in particular, he frequently demonstrated that he was feeling a sensual arousal. I use our boy hero here as the example because he shows his feelings more obviously than the female.

Play 'silly' with your imagination for a moment and imagine a line of Mums, each nursing her male offspring, and each male demonstrating this arousal with a visible erection. Imagine the offspring to be aged one year, two years, three years, and so on up to the end of the line, where the offspring is a teenager. How difficult it would be to walk along the line-up and decide at what point 'white' became 'black'. Now fortunately we do not have to make that decision at all – the little boy will make it for himself when, as Freud put it, 'he no longer mistakes the aims of his sensuality' and hurriedly points it away to the outside world. Usually he will then start to become rather 'coy' with his mother and insist on putting his pyjamas on behind the settee, and such. In one split second of time, he has torn apart two developing streams of his life; two feelings have been parted and are most unlikely to rejoin. The feelings in question are affection and eroticism.

The fact that our hero does not recall having made this immense decision fully justifies the title of a repression being given to it. (Male reader, do you remember an arousal for your mother? No, of course you don't. The memory has been repressed – but please don't be silly enough to think that you were the exception to all this, or we might have to go and ask your mother for her confirmation; and, female reader, please, please do not think that because little girls do not show it, it did not happen, because it did.)

Every one of us takes a bite from this cherry (the Oedipus complex) and every last one of us demonstrates a symptom as a result of this particular repression. **Repressions always produce symptoms.** The symptom here produced is man's inability to experience affection and eroticism at one and the same time. In fact, affection acts as a brake upon eroticism.

Look back through history and see kings of England taking the Nell Gwynnes of their time to their bedchambers; look through modern Sunday papers and read about the famous – and infamous – who take call-girls and prostitutes as their mistresses or sexual partners; look through popular fiction and see Lady Chatterley taking the gamekeeper to her bed, and if you view the phenomenon of the 'bit of rough' in the light of what we are now expounding you may understand it better.

Man feels his affection for his well-brought-up wife, who is the mother of his children, and whom he has to face at the breakfast table next morning. He feels this affection as a brake upon his eroticism; whereas, should he go with a 'woman of the streets' he will feel no such affection, there will be no brake upon his eroticism, and he will be able to indulge himself freely. On leaving her he will likely say: 'She was terrific', whereas, in fact, it was he who had been 'terrific', having achieved full potency minus the inhibiting factor of that brake.

Psychical impotence is usually construed as the proverbial 'soft half-inch in the middle' when our boy, turned man, hero finds he cannot arouse or maintain an erection. Broaden that category considerably to include premature ejaculation, inability to ejaculate whilst penetrating, frigidity and inability to climax by the female, and any other sexual malfunction you care to mention. Now look at this much broadened category of human behavioural disorder in the light of the foregoing, bearing in mind that the size of the 'bite from the cherry' will have an influencing factor, and much becomes understandable. Yet another piece to fit into our jigsaw.

I hope that by now you are coming to realize that every aspect of a person's behaviour is explainable; the fact that the person himself cannot explain it, or can only explain it erroneously, does not alter our basic belief that an effect must have a cause.

A person with a slight twitch of the eyelid will airily dismiss it with 'Oh, it's always done that', whereas we know it has only done it since the original causal factor was repressed and produced a bodily symptom. The claustrophobic will explain in great detail the awful effects upon him of going into a broom cupboard or other enclosed space. If you were silly enough to ask 'Why?', he would likely say: 'I've just told you why – because I'm claustrophobic', whereas we know an incident has been repressed, creating subconscious anxiety, which has been symbolically interpreted as a phobia. The vicar would tell us he had 'always felt a calling', but we would expect to find a cause, albeit at a subconscious level, needing the sedating effect of externalization and identification. Ask yourself how many vicars will content themselves with being right, and how many would prefer to convert you to their views. Even a person's choice of swearwords is explainable and it is certainly no accident that the anal paranoidal mentality uses 'Shit!' as an expletive and his expressions of annoyance are such as 'Oh shit and fall back on it' or something similar. Likewise the oral personality will often tone down the swear word 'bugger' to 'Oh sugar!' or similar, and 'bleeding this' and 'bloody that' are very common to our actor friend the hysteric.

Once we have accepted this dogma that any aspect of a person's behaviour can be explained, surely it is not too big a step to realize that the release of the originating repression will, as a natural consequence, remove the effect. Ah, but how to release the originating repression, that's the rub – especially as the sufferer neither knows, nor yet will willingly believe, that it is there. It sounds rather a tall order, doesn't it – and yet I help people accomplish it every working day of my life and I certainly do not class myself as a miracle worker. On the contrary, I consider every aspect of my work explainable and the results comparatively predictable, and have every hope that by the time you have fully assimilated these writings you will be perfectly capable of helping another human being to achieve a moment of 'surprising and liberating enlightenment' which is what the release of a repression brings. I say 'another human being' because, for reasons which will become clear, the only person's repressions you will not be able to release are your own – you would need the assistance of another to achieve that.

Observing at first hand the release of a repression, and witnessing the after-effects of that release, will impart that certainty of mind about the correctness of what you are doing. By the time you have a dozen or so releases under your belt you will almost certainly begin to view the time spent upon 'suggestion' therapy as time wasted, which could have been more usefully employed upon 'analytical' therapy.

5.
THE EFFECTS OF SUGGESTION

I think it's about time that we looked into (oh! if only we really could) the subconscious mind. I have alluded to it often enough, but so far without attempting to define its role in the functioning of the organism as a whole. Jung favoured the existence of an 'old' mind and a 'new' mind; and Freud was, in his later years, to amend his own theories to include various degrees of the subconscious. Here, however, we are concerned with more practical matters. I will confine myself to the facts, as I see them, and leave the dissection of infinite detail to those with the time, and the inclination, so to do.

HUMAN RECALL

This is a good time to explain that our human process of recall, particularly when assisted by hypnosis, can be in one or more of seven forms:

1. We recall an incident.
2. We recall the incident and also recall the emotion associated with the incident.
3. We recall the incident, and also recall the emotion associated with the incident, and also the bodily effect of the incident.
4. We recall the incident and the bodily affect, but not the emotion.
5. We recall only the emotion but not the incident.
6. We recall only the bodily effect but not the incident.
7. We recall the emotion and the bodily effect, but not the incident.

You often get the phenomenon of a client experiencing a

bodily sensation, for example a feeling that he was on a swing and, just as often, the arousal of an emotion – fear, sexual desire, etc., but with no intellectual explanation of the cause of that feeling or emotion. In actual fact he is of course complying with categories 5, 6 and 7 above.

When we have travelled further along this route you will begin to understand how, by the use of hypnosis, what is normally termed a 1000-hour analysis can be effectively accomplished in approximately six hours. (But remember always, that if you are going to condense and concentrate something, you shouldn't be too surprised to find that emotions, feelings, objections, approvals, fantasies, subconscious desires, resistances, etc., are all equally condensed and concentrated, and bring equally concentrated problems in their wake.) Members of the Institute of Psychoanalysis in the UK do not generally use hypnosis but rely on a more traditional, 1000-hour, analysis. Assuming we are charitable enough to rule out financial incentives from their motives, we are left to assume that their reason for using one thousand hours to do six hours' work is either they do not know how to manipulate the use of hypnosis, or they do not believe that hypnosis can bring about the desired effects – preferring complacently to accept, perhaps, Freud's dogma, that the results were 'too capricious', and so on. Once again we shall content ourselves with being right, without ever attempting to prove the other fellow wrong. I do not think I am far away from being able to prove that really hypnosis was, and is, the alchemist's stone that Freud so desperately sought, and had he but known it, he already had the key in his hand.

THE MIND AT WORK

Try to think of the human mind as a modern-day computer with different banks of memory and program interconnections. The main bank of the computer is extremely busy, having the task of carrying out something in the region of ten million processes every one-millionth part of a second – so we are told. Small wonder the main bank is little concerned with having to decide what clothes you are going to wear this morning. Nitty-gritty of that nature is left to another program bank.

We would be extremely mixed-up people if the subconscious was to waver indecisively over its functions of controlling the entire organism as a working unit, controlling as it does the entire autonomic nervous system – all the senses, hearing, seeing, touching, smelling, tasting, the respiratory system, visceral, etc. So we make a firm platform on which to begin if we state that the subconscious has no power over itself, nor yet the ability to reason: it either does – or it doesn't; it is – or isn't; it has – or hasn't. The more you think of this the more you realize that it is just as it should be. With those pressing millions of functions to carry out, the last thing we want is indecision.

There is of course an interconnection between the different parts of the mind, just as there is an interconnection between the various banks of a computer. When a clerk at regional office uses the slave unit there to input or obtain information from head-office computer, there is no awareness or visible indication at regional office of the immensely complex task being diligently performed miles away at head office. Should that same clerk try to alter the programming of the head-office master, there will almost certainly be a restriction in-built against such a happening; should that same clerk be lucky enough to succeed in bypassing that restriction and, in fact, altering the program – we could be assured the computer would now start to act upon the new information.

I think I had better finish with this particular analogy. Simply let me repeat that the subconscious – rather like that computer – has no power over itself or the ability to reason. So! If an idea does take root in the subconscious, then that idea must be discharged in motor action; and, regretfully, that rule holds good for both good ideas and bad ideas.

THE LAW OF REVERSED EFFORT

The realization that the subconscious will faithfully discharge good ideas as well as bad ideas, led Emile Coué of the New Nancy School (in practice 1905–21) to assert the proposition that where there is conflict between the imagination and the conscious will, the imagination will always win the day: 'In the conflict between the will and the imagination the force of the imagination is in direct ratio to the square of the will.' This proposition leads quite simply to what is termed 'the law of reversed effort'. When the will attempts to oppose or to command the imagination the 'law of reversed effort' applies and the will's efforts are reversed into the exact opposite. Coué used everyday examples to prove his point that if you fear an event happening, it inevitably will happen. Put a three-foot wide plank on the floor and most people could safely walk along it, but suspend the same three-foot wide plank 1000 feet up, and the reaction will be very different. The dread certainty that you are bound to fall will likely produce dire effects . . . Struggle to remember a name – the more you struggle the less likely you are to remember. Abandon your struggle and what happens? – the name is likely to spring to mind.

As a point of passing interest, the 'law of reversed effort' is the explanation of the apparent phenomenon of subjects in hypnosis experiencing physiological effects such as heaviness, lightness, eyelids 'stuck' together, hands locking – all apparently on the suggestion of the hypnotist. What in fact has happened is that when the suggestion was made the conscious will said 'That couldn't happen', the imagination said 'Aha! but it might' and in an instant of time the 'law of reversed effect' took over and ensured that the subject's eyelids stuck as firmly as if Superglue had been applied. There are other explanations of hypnotic phenomena, such as the catatonic state, but these will be dealt with later.

SUGGESTION AND THE SUBCONSCIOUS

Bernheim, in about 1882, said, 'There is no such thing as hypnosis, there is only suggestion' and his view has been compounded by many learned men since, the most insistent probably being Theodore Z. Barber. We aim to stay out of that particular argument, on the grounds that it is of theoretical interest only and has little or no effect upon the day-to-day practicalities of therapeutic endeavours. However, we do need to understand suggestion, and here we are indebted to the writings of Charles Baudoin who with Coué had created the Second Nancy School of Hypnotism. A strange choice of title for one who asserts that 'there is only suggestion', for the very word 'hypnotism' (which, incidentally, is a word I do not use) implies, I would have thought, an altered state (and sounds vaguely like an illness of some kind). I use the word 'hypnosis' instead.

Bernheim listed rules governing suggestion which are

irrefutable. When an idea takes root in the subconscious, it must be discharged in motor action or in thought: 'The idea gives birth to the idea.' Remember here that the subconscious will discharge a bad idea just as slavishly as it will a good one.

The dictionary, in defining suggestion when used as a psychiatric term, makes no allowance for the tremendous difference between auto-suggestion and hetero-suggestion, so we would be better adapting Bernheim's definition that 'suggestion is an idea which realizes itself through the subconscious mind' and that certain conditions are necessary to create auto-suggestion, i.e., the passing of a suggestion to the subconscious by oneself:

1. There must be intensity of attention to the idea itself.
2. The intensity of attention and the importance of the idea must be magnified by emotion (although it matters not which emotion is involved).
3. There must be an absence of any counter-suggestion from the psyche.

All three requirements can be met in an instant of time as a purely spontaneous thing, and indeed as part of our everyday lives, and hence suggestion is taking place constantly – with both good and bad effects upon our personality. You dread that you will be awkward and ill at ease as you walk out on to a stage – and sure enough, you are awkward and ill at ease: the idea gives birth to the idea. The suggestion, having taken root in the subconscious, discharges itself in motor action and in thought.

Just as the three requirements can be met spontaneously, so too can they be artificially created by the application of auto-suggestion during self-hypnosis. Obviously suggestion has been playing a vitally important part in your life from your earliest years. Why then do we not notice it happening? Well, think of that first requirement: the intensity of attention. That means an idea or experience so compelling that it ensnares your imagination – a sudden fear, captivating beauty, engulfing sexual desire. These, and others, will momentarily overcome, by sheer intensity, the normal barriers; but, of course, our attention being so compelled, we no longer have spare capacity to observe the phenomenon. We do it without realizing we are doing it. Once accepted into the subconscious we next tend to disavow it – after all, our only alternative would be to ascribe our most profound beliefs and emotions to some obscure and not understandable part of our mind. Oh no! Such an idea we slavishly conceal from ourselves – after all, we are only human.

Despite repeating myself so blatantly, I want to commit to print again the proposition of the idea giving birth to the idea: the conception of a vitally important subconscious process – that what takes root in the subconscious must be discharged in motor action or conscious thought. Now, however, I am going to add an important and, for our purposes, vital rider to this concept. It is this. The idea which has taken root in the subconscious wishes to be expressed. It searches unceasingly for a mode in which to be expressed, and it will be expressed, but not necessarily in its original form. It may be altered, transformed, inverted, substituted.

The idea will get realized one way or the other, but may not be recognizable as the original idea, having undergone a transformation or sublimation. In its new guise, or sublimated form, we might find ourselves giving this an entirely new name. How about – symptom? Yes, that's it, symptom.

Simply because we have been honest enough to label these altered actions or thoughts as symptoms, we cannot be so foolhardy as to expect others to follow suit. The compulsive eater is still going to say, 'Oh, it's just me, I'm greedy'; the 'hair twiddler' is going to say, 'I've always done that'; and the depressive melancholic is still going to assert, 'I've got a lot to be unhappy about.'

Nor for that matter, need we necessarily know anything about our 'symptoms'. Our subconscious is perfectly capable of making an involuntary movement without our conscious mind having the least knowledge of its existence. Chevreul, a French chemist and natural historian in the last century, recognized this fact and devised an experiment which a child can carry out, and which proves the following:

1. The subconscious can affect physical movements not under the control of the conscious.
2. The actions will be sustained by the subconscious with, without, or despite the interference of the conscious will.

3. The subconscious can be trained by repetition.

CHEVREUL'S PENDULUM

The experiment introduced above is known as Chevreul's pendulum and to do it you need the following items:

1. A piece of paper or card on which to draw a circle 40 cm in diameter, as shown in Figure 3.
2. A rod (knitting needle or similar) approximately 20 cm long.
3. A bright shiny object (wedding ring or similar) to act as 'bob weight'.
4. Approximately 20 cm of cotton to suspend the bob weight from the end of the rod.

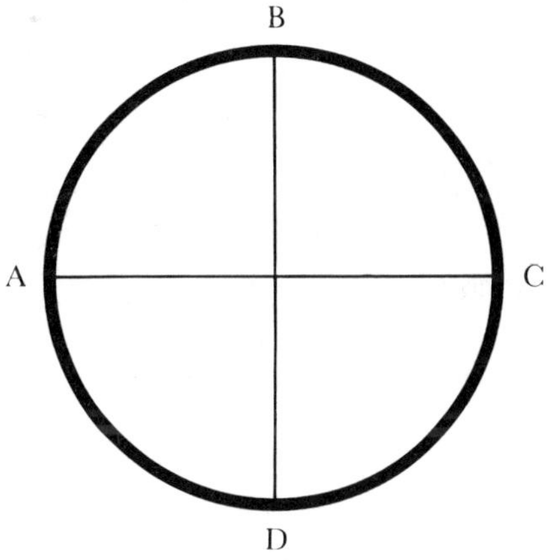

Figure 3

Now put the diagram on the floor at your feet and stand above the paper with the 'pendulum' held like a tiny fishing rod. Line up the bob with the centre cross of the diagram as you look down upon them. Now, with your hand and arm as still as you can hold them, simply concentrate on one line of the circle, say the line A–C, as you concentrate the bob weight will slowly start to swing along that line. The less you think of the bob and the more you concentrate on the line, the more the bob will swing in that direction. Change your concentration to line B–D and in due course the bob will dutifully follow. Likewise, change your concentration to the full circle

A–B–C–D and, sure enough, the pendulum will commence a circular clockwise action (anti-clockwise if you concentrate on the sequence D–C–B–A.

Repeat the whole exercise a few times and prove to yourself that, like Pavlov's dogs, your subconscious is becoming trained by repetition, and becomes more adept each time. Finally, determine to cancel the effects by intervention of your conscious will, by saying to yourself that the action will not happen – and watch yourself repeatedly fail to stop the action. Items 1, 2 and 3 of Chevreul's theory should by this time have been proved to your entire satisfaction.

In case you have not realized it, we have just about gone full circle. A few thousand words ago I said that in order to begin to understand people and their problems, you would have to understand the very cornerstone of these writings: the ability of the human mind to repress unpleasantness. In Chapter 2, I even quoted Nietzsche to help you remember it:

> 'I did this,' says my memory.
>
> 'I cannot have done this,' says my pride . . .and remains inexorable.
>
> In the end – memory yields.

Surely a repression, which is the act of concealment from ego within the subconscious, deserves to be classified as an idea taking root in the subconscious – albeit unknown to the ego of the recipient.

What do we know about the ideas that take root in the subconscious? That they must be discharged in motor action or thought – so now do you appreciate exactly why I could be so pedantic earlier on and assert so categorically that repressions always produce symtoms?

At this stage we have completed a major section of our jigsaw and you should now have some conception of what the resultant completed jigsaw puzzle will look like. (In the absence of such illumination, do not pass go, miss two throws, or move back ten squares. In other words, do not proceed until you have such insight, because it is there to be found within the writings so far.)

6.
MEETING THE CLIENT

EASE OF APPLICATION

Easy, isn't it? No, I'm not being sarcastic, I really mean it. Seriously now, isn't it all beginning to strike you as a bit too easy, just a bit too straightforward? An event or sequence of events produces a repression in a person, which as a consequence produces symptoms in that person. At a later time that person goes to a therapist, is induced into a hypnotic state and recalls, after a struggle, the original event(s) which caused the repression . . . the cathartic effect of this recall liberates the person and the symptom disappears for ever.

Once you have done this for just one person you will have 'acquired belief, the final doubt to dispel'. But it still seems too easy, doesn't it? Everything in our culture and society infers that success will come only as a result of years of study; self-denial; a fortune in development costs; an even bigger fortune in research grants; multi-million pound expenditure on drugs, diagnostic equipment, etc.

I have no intention of using these writings for any form of political platform, indeed I am almost a non-political animal. I can, however, see that Freud's dreams of hundreds of lay practitioners of psychoanalysis would in no way contribute to 'the establishment', the public school system, or the billion-pound drug industry. His observation that, 'where matters of the mind are concerned, most doctors are laymen, and that certainly includes most psychiatrists', would hardly endear him to the present-day British Medical Association. Even so, who do the media turn to for comment upon matters of the mind? Why, the doctors, of course. Many hypnotherapists and psychotherapists yearn for the approval of, and acceptance by, the medical profession. So I will declare my standpoint

I seek nobody's approval of what I do, other than my clients', and I sincerely believe that the physiological training extended to the medical profession acts as a barrier to their understanding of psychosomatic principles.

Above all things, do not let the ease of what you are doing, or rather will be doing, deceive you, and accept with resignation 'that there is no court to appeal to' – the only person who believes you is the client with whom you have just been dealing.

Imagine for a moment that you had just invented electricity and were trying to explain it to a sceptical group of listeners. Imagine the difficulties of explaining, 'You can't see it – but it will make light and heat. You can't hear it – but it will make bells ring and motors turn. You can't smell it – but it will kill you if you touch it.' Yet electric power is so easy, isn't it? In order to explain more about the human psyche, symptom formation and removal, character development and amendment, and other matters of the mind, I am going to have to switch into 'How to' language, and start talking about the practical application of what we have assimilated so far.

MEETING THE CLIENT

Assume you are in practice and somebody has sought your help to overcome claustrophobia. You patiently listen to his symptoms, bearing in mind that he is only going to tell you part of his symptoms anyway. Not forgotten already, have you? The anxiety subject, which of course the claustrophobic is, also has an inhibition in his sexual factor – he doesn't mention this, and naturally neither do you. He will usually trot out an 'erroneous association' – an incident he recalls from his younger years, which he thinks caused his claustrophobia. Here, though, a point of finite degree. It may well turn out to be the incident he describes which is at the root of his phobia, but not in the form in which he consciously recalls it. We know his association is erroneous, and not the true cause, because he's still claustrophobic – if he truly knew the cause the effect would disappear (cause and effect, remember!).

Normally, after a while, the client will falter to a stop, and look appealingly at the therapist, waiting with a dread certainty for the therapist to confirm that his horrific symptoms are far beyond the scope of any mortal therapy. Instead I just casually proceed. I want his name, age, marital status, whether a parent or not, does he smoke, does he bite his fingernails, is he prone to blushing easily, has he ever experienced an 'anxiety attack' – and here I describe it in full minus any form of title (very few people would be prepared to confirm they have had an 'anxiety attack' but most will associate with the bodily feelings and effects described). A few more simple and disarming questions. Does the person have the 'heebie geebies' about other things beside enclosed spaces, such as heights, flames, knives, rats with long tails, snakes, blood, water, death, darkness, germs, cancer . . . Here I rattle off a list for him to think about, but don't call them 'phobias'. He doesn't really view his claustrophobia as a 'phobia'; his is very special, and very peculiar to him and he's not about to admit to having any more – but he'll willingly confirm he 'couldn't pick up a spider' or the sight of blood 'makes him look away'.

Question: Does the subject find himself compulsively, and perhaps even a little foolishly, checking things – light switches, cooker knobs, car-ignition keys, house security? . . . Again, rattle off a list for him to think about. Question: Does he have a recurring dream with a very similar content to it that keeps cropping up all his life? Has he any 'ceremonial or ritual' about his daily habits? Explain that you mean something that goes way beyond just habit, and reaches almost in the realms of magic – like turning his socks inside out and back the right way again before putting them on, or washing his hands half a dozen times before breakfast.

Well now, Mr Would-be Therapist, do you think you have got enough yet to categorize your client into his character type? Of course you have! and just look at him – you do not have to read Dr Julian Faust's book *Body Language* to see what has happened. This person has relaxed. He's settled down in the chair and he's paying attention.

Now you can start to tell him things. Was it Hitler in *Mein Kampf* who said that most people do not know what they want, and that those who do know should give it to them? Well, you know you are right about this fellow; you know that his phobia is a symbolic outward interpretation of an internal anxiety – so tell him that! Wait a minute! Don't be so blunt – get him to agree that he is suffering from 'something inside himself but outside his own control'. It all means the same thing anyway, but sounds much nicer put like that. Tell him that most people who come to see you have used every ounce of their intellect upon the problem before ever walking through your door. They have puzzled over what it is that causes their stutter, or their nervous twitch, or their depression, or their anxiety, phobia, etc., etc. But despite a massive application of intellect, they still have their problem. Tell him that most people who come to see you have also used their doctor's intellect upon the problem – but they still have their problem. Tell him that most people who come to see you have also used a psychiatrist's intellect upon their problem – but they still have their problem. Did I mention to you, by the way, Mr Therapist, that you are the last resort of these people? They have been everywhere before coming to you. From doctor to psychiatrist, from homoeopath to faith healer– you name it, they've been there. So now they want 'magic'. (No, I'm not really cynical – I'm just a realist.)

Back to the client in front of you. What you are leading up to is that 'no amount of intellect is going to cure the problem', and that perhaps it is about time we stopped looking for an intellectual explanation. Your client is still nodding agreement, even though he does not fully appreciate what you are getting at. So now it is time to explain exactly what you intend to do in order to free him from his problem – it is doubtful that he will fully understand your explanation, but at least he will know what you are not going to do.

As to how to tell him, well, that is a whole different ball game. All I can do is tell you what I say; in fact, to make it easier I will talk to you now as though you were my client.

INTRODUCTORY TALK TO CLIENT

'Whenever people come to see me, with nervous twitches, stutters, depressions, anxieties, inferiority complexes, sexual problems, phobias and the like, I am never quite sure what treatment they expect – but I do know that the treatment they get is not what they had expected. That much I know for definite. I think many people have the vague idea that the hypnosis part of therapy will be all-important and that they will somehow be induced into a trance-like state where it will be put into their mind that in future they will . . . talk without stuttering . . . no longer be depressed . . . no longer be afraid of enclosed spaces . . . or whatever. In fact, Mr Client, nothing could be further from the truth. Far from putting something into your mind, in fact, something is released out of your mind, the subconscious something which had been the root cause of your particular problem.

Now I know you have probably seen stage shows, or heard of people who have had something put in their mind – if you only wanted to stop smoking I'd do that myself right now. I'd simply induce you into hypnosis, which is a very pleasant relaxed feeling, and plant post-hypnotic suggestion in your mind that you were going to stop smoking easily – and do you know, Mr Client, it would most likely happen for you just as easily as that.

Suppose, however, that you had consulted me with agoraphobia (that's a fear of going out), and just suppose I applied a similar technique. Say I planted post-hypnotic suggestions that instead of being afraid of the big open spaces, it all looked welcoming and reassuring. Take my word for it, Mr Client, rather like the smoker who was surprised to find he stopped smoking – so, too, the agoraphobic would be surprised to find he was no longer afraid of going out . . . that the open spaces did look welcoming and reassuring. Should you ask him about Mr French the therapist he would say, "wonderful – cured me of agoraphobia in one session". But, Mr Client, I wouldn't agree with him; in fact, I think Mr French should be put in prison for what he has done. (*Pause for effect.*) Cross-question that ex-agoraphobic a bit more and you may discover something rather alarming. For instance, he may no longer go in motor cars, on buses, or to the cinema . . . he has become afraid of going in enclosed spaces, or alternatively he was covered from head to foot in a nerve rash which his doctor was unsuccessfully treating as an allergy of some kind. Can you see, Mr Client, because the subconscious cause of his problem had remained – it had simply found its way out in another direction. Can you see now, why I do not plant suggestions in people's minds to remove what are obviously "symptoms"? Instead I find and remove the subconscious cause, or rather, they find and remove the subconscious cause themselves. I just show them how.

Mr Client, I want for a moment to make a comparison. It's

a bit silly, but bear with me. We've agreed that what you have really said to me is: "I have something going on inside myself but outside my own control – can you help me remove it, please?" Compare that for a moment with going to the dentist and saying, "I have a bad tooth, will you pull it out please?" The dentist says: "Yes, of course I will – open wide . . ." But every instinct in you then pulls away, you think perhaps it's not that bad after all, and you want to resist the forceps. Well, Mr Client, strange as it may sound, exactly the same is going to happen here. You are going to resist releasing that thing inside yourself every step of the way. You won't mean to, and intellectually you won't want to, and most of the time you won't even know you are doing it, but believe me – it will happen. There will even come a point where you will know you are resisting, usually about session four or five, you will likely feel it almost as a physical thing, like a wall of resistance that you are not sure that you want to go over – as though what you would find there would be awful. However, be reassured, you can go through that wall, and the other side isn't awful; in fact, it's fantastic, it's a moment of surprising and liberating enlightenment, and I aim to make sure that you reach it.

Surprising, because it comes as a complete surprise to you. You will perhaps say that you would never have believed that was in your mind. The word "liberating" speaks for itself. It sets you free – not only from your phobia but other things too that you had only thought of as behavioural pattern. Enlightenment, because you understand. You realize where your phobia really came from and with that realization comes the cure.

So that is what we are going to work for. It is not going to be easy, but there again, nor is it going to be difficult. One thing you can be sure of – it is different.

I know that when I am explaining to people at the commencement of therapy what we intend to do, I am only too well aware that it sounds impossible – that we intend to find something inside their minds that they do not know is there. However, as far as the technicalities of it are concerned, don't worry about it. I know exactly what I am doing, and I do it day in and day out, week in and week out. I already know, within certain broad guidelines, exactly how you will react during therapy – but that is merely because you are a human being and not an android. The process we use to uncover the subconscious problem is called analysis, and we carry it out with you in the hypnotic state. That, however, is the first of our difficulties, because the hypnotic state is rather ordinary and certainly non-magical. Most people would say, during and after the hypnotic experience, that it hadn't really worked for them, that they hadn't 'gone under'. It is unlikely you will feel differently, Mr Client, so please accept before we begin that the whole process will feel rather ordinary.

I expect us to take between five and eight sessions, each of approximately fifty minutes' duration and each at approximately weekly intervals. From the second session on, however, I will continually be asking you to tell me whatever comes into your thoughts. Here we come to the second major difficulty. You are going to find that the things that do come into your thoughts are things you already know about, and, disappointingly, somewhat trivial. Instead of major catastrophes in your life, you will find instead that a typical recollection is as follows: "Well, Mr French, I am only recalling when I was about thirteen, I was standing with my mum at a bus stop and I stamped in a puddle. It splashed my mother's legs and she slapped me, I felt very foolish because my friends were watching . . . that's all I was thinking of, Mr French. I'm sorry I couldn't think of anything more important." And yet, Mr Client, you will find that I appear pleased with your recollections of that tiny incident and we move on to another recollection.

By the time we get to session four you will find that you have passed over to me approximately a hundred such apparently trivial, apparently disconnected, recollections of the past, and most of them will have come from your forming years – teenage and younger. Regretfully, it is rather unlikely that you will be feeling any better as regards the problem with which you have consulted me. Indeed, you will likely find yourself feeling rather anxious – no longer so much about claustrophobia but rather more about the thought of coming here. You may possibly get an anxious feeling, as though there was something you did not want to face. Most people can fight that feeling sufficiently to make sure that they do get here, and then at session four or five you will perhaps find that an apparently abstract thought comes into your mind. Instead of a trivial recollection, you will get a thought or an impression in your thoughts, which, to you, does not seem to be real – more like imagination. At session six or seven your emotions will tell you that the thought or incident is in fact real, that it had happened and that it had been concealed within your own mind. At that point you are going to be very emotional – but you will find that it quickly subsides, that what you have realized is already becoming a matter of total indifference to you – by the next day, or thereabouts, it will have become so – and you have had your moment of surprising and liberating enlightenment.

Believable or not, that's what we are going to do, Mr Client, so can I please ask you now to lie down on the couch, just listen quietly to the sound of my voice, and we will get on with it.'

7.
THE ANALYSIS

Back now to talking to you, the reader pretending to be a would-be therapist. This is session one and things have just begun.

SESSION ONE

Now induce your client into hypnosis. Oh! I didn't explain about that! Be patient and I will – any doubts you might have about your own abilities as a 'hypnotist' I undertake to help you remove for ever before we have finished these writings.

Let us assume that you have just finished a fairly lengthy, say fifteen-minute, hypnotic induction. With the time you spent explaining things, you're now about thirty-five minutes into session one, with approximately fifteen minutes of the session remaining. Your client is lying on your consulting couch in a state of lethargic hypnosis. He has not a care in the world, his mind is relaxed, his body is relaxed, his features are in repose and he has shown you quite clearly (because you know what to look for) that he has entered the hypnotic state. (Remember, that does not mean he's gone to the planet Zod, it means he is experiencing a state of relaxation and concentration, at one with heightened awareness.)

He looks very peaceful – let us upset him! Let us use five of those remaining fifteen minutes to stir up his emotions, let him know what he is in for, prove we mean business, and just generally prepare him for session two. When we have done that, use the last ten minutes to calm him down again and to plant post-hypnotic suggestions for: (a) continuing calmness; (b) ease of recall at the next session; and (c) ease of relaxation at the next session.

So why upset him if he looks so peaceful? Well, I did say we were not in the business of suggestion therapy; we are analysts – we believe in the doctrine of cause and effect. We already know the effect, or at least a major part of it – he was only too keen to tell us that bit; now we want to know the *cause*, or, what is more to the point, we want *him* to know the cause, and you do not make omelettes without cracking eggs.

Only 50 per cent, or less, of what takes place in analysis, takes place in the consulting room; the rest takes place between sessions – and we will not even start to open any cracks in his armour until we start driving wedges in. So, here goes!

Just suggest that while he's lying here so relaxed . . . he lets his mind drift . . . wander back in time . . . back in time, as though there was no such thing as time, back into years that have gone . . . all the way back, back to his own forming, developing, impressionable years of youth, those years that brought him to maturity. Ask him to remember again, the emotions of youth, how quick to arouse, how sudden to change, to remember how he could change in an instant from loving one moment, to hating the next. Ask him to remember again the time when it was all so very new, when it was all for the first time, to remember when his own body was still a new thing and he was still finding out, and discovering, the things that he could do with it. Ask him to remember again that very first day at school, the strangeness and newness of it all. Ask him to remember changing schools to the big school, again so strange and new, and remember leaving school and starting work, just as strange, just as new.

Up to this point you have been delivering all this as a calm monologue, with little or no emotion in your voice, pausing only fractionally between incidents. You do not seek a response from him and you make this obvious by the continuity of your talk – however, you are watching. Yes, you are watching all right; every time a thought flickers through his mind you will see it registered in his features (I will save the explanation of all that to the writings about hypnosis). Now start to apply a little verbal pressure, introduce slightly more volume and charge your voice with a little emotion and proceed.

Ask him to send his mind back in those years that have gone, looking for emotion, looking for ... a storm of emotion, looking for a storm of emotion so strong and powerful, that the emotion actually penetrated the subconscious of the mind . . . so that it is still there. Ask him to look for an emotion that so troubled and so upset a young maturing mind, that the emotion is still there . . . but now . . . you want (*more loud pedal, slightly more emotion in your voice*) you want a memory, a memory of the past just to spring up into his thoughts, you want a memory just to spring up into his thoughts unbidden and unbeckoned, you want a memory just to be there in his thoughts and you want his mind to explore that memory of the past (*three-second pause and then*) and now you want his mind to link and connect, to link and to connect; one memory to another memory and you want another memory just to spring into his thoughts again unbidden, again unbeckoned – and you want his mind to explore that memory (*further three-second pause, slightly lower volume, maintain emotional charge in your voice . . . and now . . .*) you want, the very worst thing that has ever happened to him, the most emotional, the most upsetting, the worst thing that ever happened to him again, just to spring into his thoughts, not a hundred things, just one thing, the worst thing that ever happened to him and you want his mind to explore that memory (*three-second pause, lower the volume again, take the emotion out of your voice and . . .*).

Now you want him to revert to imagining things, but now when you ask him to imagine a particular thing, you want him to link the imaginary thing to something real, to something that really did happen, not necessarily anything that fits the imaginary thing, just something, a memory of something that did happen, and the first thing you want him to imagine is (*one-second pause, slight emotional charge to the voice and . . .*) water, you want him to imagine his head under water as though he was stuck underneath water, as though there was water over his nose, his eyes, his ears and his mouth, as though he was stuck underneath water (*three-second pause, then . . .*) and now you want him to imagine (*one-second pause*) pain; you want him to imagine pain that hurts, pain that really hurts and again you want him to link it in his mind to something that was real, to something that really did happen one time (*three-second pause*) and now you want him to imagine (*one-second pause*) a huge crowd of people, a huge crowd of people with everybody bigger than him, you want him to imagine himself in a huge crowd of unfriendly, unsmiling faces, with everybody bigger than him, to imagine himself lost and bewildered in the middle of a huge crowd of people, looking up at unfriendly faces, and again you want him to link this in his mind with something real (*three-second pause and . . .*) now you want him to imagine the opposite (*one-second pause*), you want him to imagine a lonely place where there's only him, as though he was the last person left in the whole world, a lonely place where there is nobody else, as though there was only him, completely alone, and again you want him to link it in his mind with something that was real (*three-second pause and . . .*) finally you want him to imagine (*one-second pause*) flames, you want him to imagine flames everywhere, as though the world was on fire, flames that won't go out, flames everywhere, you want him to imagine flames burning, and once again you want him to link it in his mind to something that really did happen (*three-second pause and then . . .*).

Now, just as you have asked him to imagine things and link them in his mind to real things, now . . . you are going to accuse him of certain things, but when you accuse him of these things, you don't want him to think 'Oh, no, I didn't do that', you want him instead to link merely it all in his mind to something that really happened – not necessarily anything that fits the accusation, but just something, a memory, something that really did happen . . . and, the first thing you are going to accuse him of is (*one-second pause . . .*) having a guilty secret, a guilty secret that he doesn't want you to know about, a guilty secret that he'd prefer not even to think about, you're going to accuse him of having a guilty secret, and again you want him to link this in his mind to a memory, a memory of something that did happen (*three-second pause*) and now . . . you are going to accuse him that (*one-second pause*) when he was only a young fellow, back in those younger years of his life, when he was only a youngster, that one time he showed himself up, embarrassed himself so much he just wanted the ground to open up and swallow him, that one time he showed himself up, embarrassed himself so much he just wanted the ground to swallow him up, and again you want him to link it in his mind to a real memory (*three-second pause*) and finally you want to accuse him (*one-second pause*) that back in those young years, when he was only a young lad, there was this grown-up man, this grown-up man, and he let this grown-up man touch him, interfere with him, that he let this grown-up man touch him and now you want a person to spring into his thoughts, and stay in his thoughts, you want a person to spring into his thoughts and stick there (*three-second pause*) but now . . . you want him to stop thinking about the past, you want him to start thinking about today (*here revert back to a quiet, calm monotone*). You want him to relax and be calm . . . and now you use up the remaining minutes of the session to calm him down and to lodge post-hypnotic suggestions aimed at assisting your therapeutic endeavours – of which more later when we discuss hypnosis.

I am going to explain what exactly we have done in that first session I have just described, and why we have done it. But first I want to issue a timely warning: we are only part-way into these writings, and if somebody was giving you directions to find a small village in Wales, and got as far as saying, 'You go first of all to Bristol', I am sure you would agree that you would be somewhat lost when you got to Bristol if you had not even waited to find out the name of the village in Wales you were looking for, let alone the remaining directions to find it.

In case my sarcasm escapes you, I will tell you a true story, of events that happened in my consulting room not long ago. A lady client, aged about 38 years, consulted me with migraine headaches and a phobia of some kind, I cannot remember what. She was no more than averagely responsive to the hypnotic state, and I proceeded pretty well as I outlined in the preceding pages, just as I have done many hundreds of times before, and just as I have done many hundreds of times since. But, in her case, when I got as far as asking her to remember the worst thing that happened to her, she started to get extremely distressed, her breathing became extremely rapid and her face flushed, her face continued flushing but the breathing almost stopped. She appeared to have difficulty breathing and was clutching at her throat. She tore from her neck a string of beads and tore the neck of her jumper. Her eyes were closed but started to protrude from her head, her neck started to shrink in size, her face turned purple, and then almost black, her tongue swelled and protruded from her mouth. She was obviously desperate for air and was still tearing her hands at an 'imaginary' ligature around her neck. The whole incident lasted about three minutes and at one stage her neck was so constricted that its diameter was little more than a drinking cup – as an aftermath to the incident her neck was quite badly bruised and swollen. Now that's what is called an abreaction: in her case she was abreacting (reliving with emotion and physical effects) an incident where her father had, literally, attempted to strangle her with a leather belt when she was about eleven years old.

Now, unless you feel ready to deal with such an incident, do not go putting the 'how to' part of my writings into practice. Be patient. Wait awhile. One thing a successful therapist – particularly an analyst – must have is restraint.

There is a purpose behind that first session. At the outset of these writings I asked you to cease viewing hypnosis as an end-product, but rather as the beginning to something else. Hypnosis gives easier, but not necessarily easy, access to the more hidden thoughts and emotions, and allows a much greater state of rapport between therapist and client; the critical faculty of the subject is somewhat withdrawn and his usual inhibitions considerably relaxed. He will listen too, and often accept without criticism, many comments that in his everyday state he would view as silly, offensive, distasteful, imaginative, and so on.

Let us assume that our subject had a distressing experience in the swimming baths at an earlier age – where the emotions, connected to being under water, had been repressed, but not the memory. That emotion wants releasing; otherwise it is going to interfere with analysis proper. Unreleased, that emotion will dictate the course of the first couple of sessions by repeatedly bringing thoughts of swimming, face-washing, choking, etc., into the subject's conscious thought patterns. Far better to have it out, just like a bad tooth, at the outset. The wording of that first session 'dig', aims at likely upsets of youth. Many people will be untouched by all of it, but a higher percentage, certainly more than half of your clients, will feel a wave of emotion at one of your arrows.

The first session to which we have just submitted our client, had other purposes besides just attempting to clear extraneous emotion out of the way. We have started a process of recall which will now be an ongoing rolling ball, gathering size and momentum as it rolls. During the interval between sessions, our client will have all sorts of little stray memories from his past literally 'pop up' in his thoughts. When he sits quietly watching TV, he will suddenly find his attention has wandered and a recollection from his youth has presented itself to his consciousness. When you see him the next week he may say something like: 'I've been thinking hard as I can all week, but I'm afraid I haven't come up with anything really important.'

Realize at this point that the wording of the first session was such that it also took the form of 'post-hypnotic suggestion' for recall. The client also knows that you are in charge, that you are positive in your approach, positive in what you are going to do, and positive in the way you are going to do it. Goodness knows, he hardly got a word in edgeways; he had no sooner started to elaborate his symptoms then you politely shut him up and got him to agree it was all 'inside himself, but outside his own control' – and straight away started laying down what was going to happen. In his heart of hearts he quite likes this – it is nice to hand over to someone else. It had been hard for him to admit to himself he needed help at all, but once that decision was taken, it was nice to be taken in charge. The phenomenon of transference has begun. Freud recognized this and said he wanted to make it clear that transference exists from the beginning of the therapy. We see no sign of it. We need not reckon with its existence – yet.

SESSION TWO

When your client walks back through the door for his second session, in the first instance it is you again who wants to be doing all the talking, otherwise your client is only going to produce a load of intellectual resistance. I have found it very good policy to use, at the first session, one of the commercially available psychological tests, such as the Carver test or the Lüscher test. The one I usually use is the Lüscher test, which is based on a random selection of eight different colour codes. Amazingly simple to administer, it takes less than two minutes of session time. During the week between sessions I write out about a foolscap page of the client's 'psychological profile' as interpreted by the test, which is mostly penetratingly accurate. At the commencement of the second session, after a short preamble, I read this profile out to the client. This has a twofold purpose:

1. He is reassured that my apparent disinterest in his symptoms was excusable, as I seemed to know an awful lot about him anyway and had obviously given thought to him, subsequent to his visit.
2. My apparent perception of his wishes and desires in life will impress that it would be rather pointless to attempt to conceal his true nature as I have obviously seen through his normal façade.

I would not normally ask my client to comment as to whether he thought the profile was accurate, but many clients will do so unprompted. The vast majority of the time they are amazed at the penetrating accuracy, and will often say so.

Now I again ask him to lie on the couch and relax. I carry out a five-to seven-minute induction into the hypnotic state, and then ask him again to let his thoughts drift back into his past, and I stress words such as 'intensity of experience' and 'intensity of emotion'. I ask him to gather a memory into his thoughts and then say: 'And now I'd like you to tell me exactly what you find yourself thinking about now.' . . . and I wait . . . Should they not speak within ten seconds, I prompt: 'Go on, tell me whatever you're thinking about at the moment.' Nine times out of ten (I will discuss the tenth one at a later time) the person will produce a small recollection of some comparatively trivial 'psychological experience' of the past. I use the expression 'psychological experience' rather than the word 'memory' because if he has not told you what it meant to him at the time, then he has not really told. A person saying, 'I am recalling being at the dinner table at about age eight' will not suffice, but if the same subject says, 'I am recalling being at the dinner table at about age eight and I was jealous because my brother got a larger portion than me' then he has satisfied the requirements of analysis.

The moment the person comes to a pause, I jump in and say, 'Fine, the thoughts of that meal table I want you to link in your thoughts, connect in your mind, and now I want you to tell me whatever you find yourself thinking about.' The next recollection is most unlikely to appear to be connected in any way, shape or form to the first one. But again, at the pause, I use the same expressions of link and connect in order to goad another recollection from his thoughts. When he has produced about four recollections, I then explain that I want him to do it all alone now, without me speaking. I say that I want him to wait in the blankness of his thoughts until he finds an impromptu recollection presenting itself, and then to recount it – when he comes back to a blankness, to await another impromptu recollection and to repeat it without comment from me. When he has 'gone solo' for a few recollections, one may well crop up which is of a sexual nature: after he has introduced the subject of sexuality, I interrupt during one of his blanks, and say, 'Fine, thank you very much, and now I want you to relax again and just listen quietly to my voice – but while I'm talking I want you to be darting your memory back into the past, seeing if you can't find little recollections which vaguely fit what I am saying.' I go on to explain that some of what I say may well appear childish but I further explain that I go through this with everybody. Then I dwell upon the genital period of development; using pretty well the same words as I used earlier in these writings when I discussed childhood realization of the 'difference' between the sexes, the differing effect upon us all, the confusion on the subject of 'blood' and the silly explanation of why boys and girls are different. I take pause for effect at various points within the discourse and I am constantly watching for reaction within the client. At the end of that I simply say, 'But that's all just part of growing up. I want you merely to send your memory back amongst those years and just tell me the first thing you find yourself thinking of.' From then to the end of the session I get the client to keep using the process of free association to recount memory after memory.

Again, at the end of the session, when he opens his eyes and sits up, I bid him good-day as quickly as is politely possible and try to avoid any intellectual discussion of the session content.

He has now had what I mentally call his 'bridge-crossing session' where he has actually started to impart anecdotes from his life. He has well and truly realized that it is not going to be as simple a matter as dropping in the doctor's for a prescription; in fact his recovery is going to require time, money, effort – and self-discipline – on his behalf.

I will discuss the recalcitrant client, and the many possible vagaries likely to appear as resistance to our work, at a later time; for now I am going to continue explaining how I proceed in a rather stereotyped manner with Mr Average.

Pursuant to session two the client is going to find that the incidence of 'chance recall' becomes more marked during the week. As the client pauses for a break at his office desk his mind will wander and some little incident from his past is likely to appear in his thoughts. I do not think I have made it clear, but at this stage, for the first two to three weeks of analysis, our hero usually does feel the better for having consulted us. He is not about to say so, though, for reasons I have previously expounded; but for all that, he is feeling calmer and the intensity of his symptoms are being toned down. I steer well clear of any discussions about that though, and if the subject crops up, I simply remind him that it is the end-result that we are looking for and not some minor interim improvement. However, 'such fine weather cannot last forever' and in the making of our proverbial omelette we still have many eggs to crack.

SESSION THREE

Once again, the sooner your client is on the consulting room couch and hypnotized the better. Inconsequential chatter at the start of the session should be kept to the bare minimum, whilst at the same time one should be wary of appearing curt or short. It is worth mentioning here that you cannot even comment upon the weather without your client looking for innuendoes in what you have said. 'I wonder, was he trying to tell me something?' will often go through his thoughts. This is because the phenomenon of transference is already well established; indeed, having been present from session one, it is now gathering strength and, although we as yet see no sign of it and as yet need not concern ourselves with its existence, it is already playing a vitally important role in the progress of the analysis. The explanation of transference is a lengthy and complicated one and although transference is the subconscious motivation allowing the analysis to proceed to a satisfactory conclusion, I shall save my explanation until I start talking about obstacles, difficulties, resistances and the like. This is because, although it may appear a paradox in terms, the thing which motivates the analysis forward is also the most likely thing to bring it to a stop.

I suspect that, like myself, you will only finally come to believe in the correctness of what you are doing, with that certainty of belief 'the final doubt to dispel', when you have observed the phenomenon of transference at first hand, time after time – *ad infinitum.*

In an ideal third session the therapist should just do a three- to five-minute induction into the lethargic state of hypnosis and then simply ask the client once again to let his mind wander back into the past and to say out loud the first thing he finds himself thinking of; thereafter the client should only be prompted if he runs dry but otherwise should simply proceed from recollection of one incident to recollection of another incident, to another, and so on. In my own mind I call the third session the 'involvement' session, because most times, that is just what it does – it involves him, he gets totally caught up in it and finds the net of analysis is widening to encompass even more aspects of his life. I do not honestly think it is too much of an exaggeration to say that before analysis is complete the client will feel as though it has called into question his very right to exist.

Session three is the real spadework of the analysis and much ground should be turned over. The session is quite likely to have a deep effect upon the emotions of the client during the week between sessions, but I did say fine weather couldn't last forever, didn't I?

I want you now to grasp what is actually happening in the analysis. Well, first and foremost, the client's ego is being trained not to take flight and run away from things – to take off the rose-tinted spectacles. Ask me what my army service was like and I will likely reply, 'Fine, enjoyed every minute of it.' Get me pinned down and cross-question me, and before you know it I will be talking of monsoon ditches overflowing, tents that leaked, comrades injured or killed, homesick 5000 miles away, and so on. What price that 'Fine, enjoyed every minute of it' now?

Secondly, the client is getting used to 'transferring' things across to the analyst – it is true to say that the responsibility for the whole problem and the curing of the problem has been transferred from the client to the analyst.

Thirdly, and just as important, the client has been persuaded to stop applying his intellect to the problem. In the process of 'free association' he is particularly requested, nay! entreated, No! demanded, to say whatever comes into his thoughts. It has been stressed that it matters not whether the thought appears ridiculously trivial, indeed whether it appears totally irrelevant, or whether the thought is somewhat shameful or whether the thought in his mind had been previously viewed as a secret. We have made this our only true rule or condition of treatment. We want the client to abide by that single fundamental rule that he will say whatever comes into his head: if he does this, we can help him; if he does not, or cannot, then we cannot help him.

Should I not have been able to get the client into this state of 'co-operation' by, say, midway through session three, then I would likely stop the session and discharge him from treatment – but I will elaborate upon such difficulties at a later time.

Because we use the hypnotic phenomenon, our sessions are having far more effect between times than ever conventional analysis could hope for – and this, of course, is the reason why we are so dramatically speeding up the process. Should you have delved deeply into Freud's writings you will have discovered that he professed to have abandoned the use of hypnosis for reasons which he never made outwardly clear, although he does admit to doubts as to his own abilities as a hypnotist; he also speaks of results obtained being 'capricious' and there is certainly no doubt that he was tremendously affected by the lady client whose 'transferences' within the hypnotic state, caused her at session end to clasp 'Sigis' to her bosom professing her love for ever. Whatever the reasons, he decided to dispense with 'it'. Interestingly enough, I don't think he ever did – I think he only thought he did. What do I mean? Well, I don't think for one moment that the use of hypnosis is confined to so-called 'hypnotists'; it is as much a part of our everyday life as breathing or eating. Read, for example, Dr Donald J. Moine's dissertation on the use of hypnotic language within the selling profession, and you will see that I am not alone in believing that many people use hypnosis without even realizing that they are doing so, and without those at the receiving end ever being aware that the phenomenon was involved.

I make no apologies for interposing at this point the fact that I do not think James Braid (1795–1860), who first coined the word 'hypnosis' and who borrowed from the Greek so to do, deserves any medals for having used such a word. He was himself to come to the realization of his error, and tried to substitute the word 'monoedism', but he was too late, the title had caught hold.

I myself profess the title 'hypnotherapist' for one reason, and one reason only: as a hypnotherapist, I get clients flocking to me; as a 'psychotherapist', or as a 'psychoanalyst' I would get very few. There is a social stigma attached to psychological treatment and anything which smacks of it, but hypnotherapy is socially acceptable (well, slightly – at least more than the others). As a point of interest, I am listed in the telephone directory's *Yellow Pages* under both Hypnotherapist and Psychotherapist and I average around two thousand enquiries a year for my services as a hypnotherapist, and around two or three enquiries a year as a psychotherapist. No need for cynicism – just accept it. Was it not St Francis of Assisi who wanted 'the courage to change the things that he could change; the serenity to accept the things that he couldn't change; but above all, the wisdom to know the difference between the two'?

I'm confident in my own mind that Freud did continue using hypnosis long after he thought he had abandoned it. His techniques involved a warm room, isolated from outside noises, and free from distractions; to position himself behind, and consequently out of sight of, the subject; to cause the client to close his eyes; and sometimes to apply a focal point of attention to the client's forehead by applying pressure with the heel of his palm. That is enough to cause any sceptic to go into hypnosis, but, since there is no such thing as a hypnotized feeling, the subject would not realize, and since the observable phenomenon of the hypnotic state needs trained eyes to detect, neither would the 'accidental hypnotist'.

Hypnosis, and therapies associated with it, have gone in and out of fashion like yo-yos over the years, and, if you will forgive the rather vulgar analogy, the participants are rather like the teenage girl who thinks she 'is the only one who has got one' or the teenage boy in his discovery of sex who thinks he 'invented it'.

The year 1981 saw much publicity given to a six-hour operation, involving major abdominal surgery, carried out utilizing hypnoanaesthesia. The subject was a 24-year-old woman in Pennsylvania, USA, the surgeon one Dr J.S. Lapcevic and the hypnotechnician a Myrna J. Morris. Without detracting in any way from their contribution to our understanding, it would pay to remember that Dr James Esdaile (1808–59) carried out thousands (yes, thousands) of major surgery operations utilizing the same process before the middle of the nineteenth century. To think that well over a century has gone by, with no significant advances being made in that direction, does not really extend much hope for immediate future happenings, does it. Present public interest in alternative medicine is psychologically explainable, just as a neurosis is explainable, and the factors which go to make that explanation are, rather like a neurosis, not fixed and squared off, but a constantly growing and changing thing.

We certainly do use hypnosis and we understand thoroughly the subconscious forces at work. Our client has no conception of the forces at work within him, and from that point of view can be likened to a lamb to the slaughter. Fortunately, we are not out to slaughter him, but simply to bring him to a resolution of his problem – although I suspect that, before we have finished, he may well have cause to question that.

Let us assume now that we have had an averagely good session three – that the client has used the process of free association to expound about fifteen or twenty recollections from his past and has kept his intellectual intrusion to a minimum. Once again, at the end of the session, we should encourage him to depart fairly soon after concluding the hypnotic state and avoid, again as far as possible, too much discussion. At the same time, it is good to be reassuring, and if the client is behaving and responding as you would wish there is no harm in saying so, and confirming that, as far as you are concerned, the whole thing is proceeding on the course you require, and that you can see no reason for his 'moment of surprising and liberating enlightenment' not arriving on schedule. Here I will add that I never lie to clients: should the truth be unpalatable I attempt, if necessary, to avoid it, but that is as far as I go. Nobody, but nobody, can ever throw back at me, 'But you said . . . so and so . . .'. If I said it, I meant it, and would be able to reiterate why.

When the client leaves after session three the 'between-session' activity of his mind is going to be greater and there is a strong chance that before session four he will come to a major, internal and unconscious, hurdle. What this means for him, and for you, I will leave until I discuss the difficulties in detail, for now I will confine myself to talking about the 'less problematical' client, representing slightly more than half of the people who consult.

SESSION FOUR

There is every chance that the client will be feeling vaguely anxious when he presents himself for session four. You are likely to see him view the consulting couch as an alien hostile planet, and plonk himself in a more formal discussion chair prepared to talk on any subject under the sun rather than proceed with the analysis. When you observe these things, it is good to be rather teasing and light-hearted about it – but nevertheless to get him on that couch at all costs. 'All animals are equal, but some animals are more equal than others,' said Orwell. Well, likewise with our sessions – all sessions are equally important but some are more equally important than the others. Tease, reassure, ask and tell, but get him on the couch, and get him in hypnosis. Restart the process of free association after a cursory three- to five-minute induction and allow him to proceed unhindered for about ten minutes or so.

At this stage I use a technique based on 'automatic writing' principles, which I explain in Chapter 9: An Introduction to Hypnosis. The technique simply involves a post-hypnotic suggestion, requiring the client to write down a reason for his anxiety. The suggestion I give makes it clear that the person is to write something down at the end of the session. Having given the suggestion, I then ask the client to recommence using free association and to continue verbally relating whatever comes into his thoughts. Through to the end of the session I keep him to his pact of recounting whatever does come into his thoughts.

At the end of the session I wait for him to write something down for me, and then once again I speedily bid him good-day.

SESSION FIVE

By this stage, the majority of clients are somewhat despondent about the potential efficacy of our therapy. I suspect that one of the more trivial of the many, many reasons why analysis has never 'caught on' as a popular therapy has to do with our welfare state, as I fear that many clients who had no financial involvement in their analysis would withdraw at this point. Our client already has a 75 per cent investment in his recovery, though, and is reluctant to throw that away, so here he is for session five.

Yet again the session should be got under way as soon as possible. Following a three- to five-minute induction, the client should again use the process of free association to impart recollections from his mind.

You will have noticed that I talk of three- to five-minute inductions each time, after the first and subsequent session. When you have learnt more about hypnosis you will perhaps wonder why I use that amount of time and self-effort to achieve something that can often be effected with just one click of the fingers. Well, there are very few things I do in my consulting room that do not have a reason behind them, and this is certainly not one of them. As you learn to study hypnosis more and more, you will become aware of the 'Pavlov's Dogs' effect – the fact that the subconscious can be trained by repetition and can be programmed for future action by post-hypnotic suggestion. Effectively, at the end of session one, you could say to the subject in hypnosis, words to the effect that, next time he saw you . . . simply the click of your fingers . . . the click of your fingers – and you demonstrate by clicking your fingers – will cause him to relax into hypnosis. Should the idea take root in the subconscious then it must be discharged in motor action, which means that if your suggestion has been sufficiently well worded, then that is all it would take at session two – simply ask the subject to lie back and relax . . . and then merely click your fingers. To save your subject a lot of embarrassment during the week following that first session, it would be sensible to make sure that your suggestion contained instruction that it was to be only the click of your fingers and not other clicks, and only in your presence – otherwise the client is going to feel rather foolish after somebody snaps his fingers for the waiter in his favourite restaurant!

So, why do I wear out my long-suffering vocal chords with a more lengthy induction each time? Well, in a word – empathy. Remember, I am not in the least interested in proving anything to do with hypnosis, there is no test of one-upmanship, there is no conflict, there is no question of a superior mind dominating the client's mind; there are only two people working together in harmony to achieve a therapeutic aim. You are asking this man to 'bare his soul' – to lay before you the most intimate thoughts of his life, and he will do that – not with dominance, not with coercion, but with empathy, with transference (that word does keep cropping up, doesn't it). Here, at session five, he is not all that far away from the ultimate sacrifice of all. To submit him to even the most minor indignity of a finger-snapping technique or key-word induction can only have a harmful effect upon that empathy.

The closer and closer I get to explaining the end of analysis, the forces at work during and after the analysis, the mechanism of cure which takes place, and the therapeutic aim which will have been achieved, the more dismayed I become at the near impossibility of the task; not doing it – explaining it! Had I taken each of my readers through analysis it would then require little or no explanation; I could confine myself more to the technicalities involved.

I am reminded that the last time a crippled person walked out of my consulting rooms after ten years or so in a wheelchair, it got front page publicity locally under the heading 'Miracle'. But the attitude of a disbelieving public is summed up by what a radio news reporter said when interviewing me about it. He believed he had explained the phenomenon to his own satisfaction with the word 'psychosomatic': 'It was all in her mind – she wasn't really crippled at all and really you the therapist didn't do anything for her she couldn't have done for herself at any time, by shaking herself out of it.'

I wonder how many times the claustrophobic has been told to 'shake himself out of it' at the entrance to a lift; how many times the depressive has been told to 'shake himself out of it' and cheer up; how many times the migraine sufferer has been told to 'shake himself out of it, it's only a headache'; and so on; the examples are innumerable.

Ponder on this for a moment: as a result of analysis with me, usually averaging between five and eight sessions, dozens of ex-migraine sufferers no longer have a hint of migraine, no matter what they eat; dozens of ex-stutterers no longer stutter, no matter what stress they are subjected to; many ex-claustrophobics can go into cinemas, broom cupboards, motor cars or any enclosed space; plenty of ex-psychically impotent males and females are living a happy and exciting sex life; numerous compulsive eaters are slim without recourse to diet; dozens of ex-anorexics are eating a healthy diet. I had better stop or it will sound like megalomania, and if there was any conceit involved, I would not wish to commit it to print. I am simply stating facts, and, again, contenting myself with knowing that I am right. I appreciate that I was only the catalyst and that the people effected their own cures, so the question of conceit or self-satisfaction does not really arise. What I am trying to do is to explain the enormity of the problem – not the curing of it, but the explaining of the curing of it, and if I am having difficulty with you, dear reader, imagine how difficult it is with a client.

Should just one doctor, anywhere in the world, totally cure just one case of migraine, he will almost certainly become world-famous, and his treatment, in all probability will be named after him. The ex-cripple I have just mentioned – had that been carried out by delicate surgery or wonder drugs, it would have received world-wide recognition, and the physician invited on lecture tours, etc.

Our therapy, on the other hand, concerns that which is most intimate in a person's thoughts – it effects an internal change in the subject, and, although he will be suitably grateful for your intervention, he is not about to, nay cannot, disclose what took place to bring about that change.

You will have noticed from the foregoing that riches and fame are most unlikely to be your lot via the use of analysis. You are far more likely to attract the attention of the media should they see a chance to grant you the recognition of notoriety. All we can do now with our disillusioned client at session five is to keep him at it; he is not far away from releasing his subconscious anxiety, though as far as he is concerned it could be on the moon, he thinks his chances of finding it are so remote.

As the session progresses one particular thought will often keep recurring: 'I keep thinking a lot of that dining room at our old house' would be a typical comment. By about halfway through the session his thoughts will be almost dominated by one focal point – although his mind will still keep drifting away to other things, and typical comments will be, 'It's as though I was looking at it on film'; 'I can't seem to think of anything else except that . . .'.

At this stage the client is more likely to experience a physical phenomenon too, a peculiar feeling of some kind. Again, typical comments would be, 'I have the silliest feeling. I feel as though I'm rolling off the couch – but I know I'm not' or, 'I feel as though I'm spinning round and round' or, 'I feel very excited and anxious' or, 'I feel sexually aroused but cannot explain why'. Before the end of the session he is likely to get in his thoughts an 'impression', a sort of apparently imaginary thought or picture, so a typical spoken comment would be, 'I have the silliest picture in my mind' or, 'I can see my dad standing over me with a raised stick . . . but he never hit me, I wonder why I'm imagining that.'

Now it is imperative that the client be cajoled into saying out loud whatever he is thinking, fantasizing, feeling. An idea is going to present itself to his consciousness, but that idea is likely to be repugnant to him or, alternatively, to represent a complete reversal of what he has always believed. When the therapist speaks it should be in an emotionally charged, expectant voice, giving suggestions such as: 'Tell me the next thing that happened, the next thing, the very next thing' and also, 'It's all right to remember, it's perfectly all right to remember, what troubled a young mind will be all right to a grown mind – it's all right to remember.' Bear in mind the fact that the subject is in hypnosis so we are hoping for these suggestions to lodge in the subconscious.

Most often session five will fizzle out like a damp squib and the person will leave rather puzzled and confused. Just as often, there will be an idea whirling around his thoughts as to what it could be that we are looking for. The thought may not only be repugnant to him, but may also appear to be apparently incredible, possibly a complete reversal of what he has always believed. (He has a full week to stew over all that, though.)

SESSION 6

Properly handled, session six can be the conclusion to analysis; mishandled, it can leave you with a long haul ahead.

The presenting client is almost certain to be in a high state of internal resistance by now. During the intervening week, the focal point of his thoughts will have been intellectualized, and firmly discounted. Do not mention it, don't ask him how he has been, just say hello and get on with it. Let good manners and politeness, if necessary, take second place, and very breezily assert, 'Come on then, on the couch, and let's get on with it; time presses.' Stall all attempts at conversation, just get him onto the couch and into the hypnotic state.

Now this is where you have got to be patient. For the first twenty minutes or so of the session the client's mind will likely continue the process of free association. Take my word for it, at the back of his thoughts, last week's 'idea' is still hovering – but, if you are the one to mention it, then you are the one who 'put it into his thoughts'. Wait . . . he will come back to it, and when he does – pounce! Get after his emotions – it was emotion that repressed this complex and it will be emotion that releases it, so demand emotion from him. Charge your own voice with emotion and suggest in a very powerful tone that what he experienced then he is to experience again now . . . that what emotions he felt then he is to feel again now . . . that what physical sensations he experienced then he is to experience again. The empathy and transference between client and therapist is now so total he will excuse you anything! You can shout at him, accuse him, harangue him – but make him remember. He will do it for you if you demand it of him. So demand it, and keep demanding it until, in a flurry of emotion 'it' all comes back into his mind – his moment of surprising and liberating enlightenment has arrived. A few more words, and you can sit back and relax. Scrawl on the back of his notes 'Repression released – case closed'. Let your client bring his emotions back under control and he can leave – he has an insight into himself few other people possess. He knows now that 'things' do not 'just happen' at all. Nothing at all happens unless all the prerequisites have been fulfilled. This world is really a very orderly place where things happen according to strict universal laws and we unconsciously contribute to the prerequisites all the time. For every effect there is a cause, and our client now knows the causes of his effects – his symptoms are disappearing by the second.

To explain analysis even more fully I will go through an actual case roughly as it happened.

EXPLANATORY CASE STUDY – A STUTTERER

Male, mid-thirties, single; consults with speech impediment – a stutter – which he has had since the age of 9 years. Comes particularly when under stress. Initial interview reveals the following: he smokes, bites his fingernails, is very predisposed to blush and he declares his sexuality to be hetero – adding that he has remained unmarried because Miss Right has so far eluded him.

The first session was uneventful, following the standard pattern I have previously outlined. Session two was equally uneventful and, in fact, it took a lot of effort and haranguing to get him to begin disclosing his thoughts. He was frequently to assert that his mind was blank – interrogation proved he was committing the cardinal sin of holding back thoughts because 'they were too trivial to mention'. However, by the start of session three he had caught on to what was required and lay as good as gold in the lethargic state of hypnosis, with his eyes closed, disclosing the free associations that came into his mind as follows:

1. I am just thinking of our back garden at home, my dad had cut the hedges in the shape of birds – I used to run around under them.
2. Now I'm thinking how me and my friends used to sit on a white wall at the bottom of the road – there was an orchard we weren't supposed to go in.
3. Now I'm riding my bike down the road, a friend waiting on the corner. A bloke had taken my friend's bike off him

but we got it back.

4. A much bigger boy down the road used to bully me a lot – I told my dad in the end. He said 'Stand up for yourself.' I did and it stopped.
5. I had a friend called Alice. We played every day together, but then Dad said we might be moving and I told her. I started thinking to myself I'd have no friends at all if we moved.
6. One time it was dusk and we were still running up and down on our bikes. Mum got very cross and kept shouting to come in.
7. When I was learning to swim, Dad used to take me. I had some little red swimming trunks and he'd hold these at the back and his other arm under my chest to teach me.
8. I keep getting an impression of my old road in the half dark – can just see the shape of the houses.
9. We all used to congregate round that white wall at the bottom of the road of an evening, swapping football cards and things like that.
10. That white wall was up by the main road – behind it was all trees and bushes and dark places – I didn't like it very much. I wasn't supposed to go in there anyway.
11. One time there was a man standing by that white wall in a brown suit. Don't see why I should think of him, though.
12. By that white wall was some spare ground we used to play on a lot, and next to it was a house where the man kept telling us to go away 'cos we made too much noise.
13. I'm thinking of that man in the brown suit again, by that white wall and I have the most peculiar feeling that I ought to know something about him – but I haven't the slightest idea what.
14. Now I'm simply thinking of sitting on the side of the road on a nice day in summer, just day-dreaming.

At that point of session three I carried out a sequence from 'automatic writing' technique (discussed in Chapter 9). As he sat up at the session end he wrote on the paper as follows: 'I am going home now.'

His only comment was to remark that the writing looked

more like his schoolday's writing than today's. Had I asked him, which of course I didn't, for an intellectual explanation of what he had written, then on the preponderance of probabilities, he would have said something to the effect that it was the end of the session and consequently time to go home. However, I didn't ask him. I simply gathered up the paper and politely wished him good-day.

Session four started off comparatively uneventfully but, by degrees, developed until it brought the analysis to an early, and very successful, conclusion. The following represents the sequence of recall:

15. I'm seeing again the shape of our old road, the houses, the white wall at the end and the trees behind it.
16. I'm just thinking of being on my own and walking across that spare ground. I was about nine years old.
17. Now I'm just thinking of sitting on that white wall. I'm sorry, I just don't seem able to think of anything else.
18. I'm remembering that one time I did climb over that wall and go scrumping apples from the trees.
19. I recall sitting on the ground under the trees eating apples.
20. My mind just flashed to that man in the brown suit, but I don't know why.
21. I know when I was sat on the ground eating apples I could see the man through the branches – he was on the other side of the wall.
22. Thats funny! I don't remember this, but I can imagine that man climbing over the wall; it's like seeing it on film.
23. I can imagine him walking through the trees. I'm sure I'm not really remembering this, though.
24. It's just as though he was searching round in the trees and I was trying to hide from him sat on the ground.
25. I can just see the man standing there. Oh! This doesn't make sense . . . he's undoing his trousers.
26. I'm beginning to feel very anxious. I'm also beginning to think that this could be real and not imagination. I feel very anxious, in fact frightened. I think we might have to stop this session soon.
27. It seems to be more and more real: he's masturbating in

front of me. I was really frightened, I wanted to get away. He's saying something to me – I was kneeling on the grass – he's moving closer and closer.

28. I said to him 'I don't like this – I'm going home now' and tried to run past him, but he grabbed me. He grabbed my shirt and he's trying to get my trousers down.
29. He got me pinned down on the grass and was half-standing over me – trying to sit on me. I was moving my head from side to side. He's trying to hold my head with one hand and masturbating in front of my face with the other.
30. He's pulling my hair and pressing it against my lips – trying to force my mouth open. He's taken his hand out of my hair and forcing my mouth open with his fingers. I'm trying to shout and throwing my head from side to side. (By this stage the client was extremely emotional and sexually aroused.)
31. I can actually feel it now, it's on my lips, he's rubbing it on my face, ugh! He's come, he's wiping it round my face.
32. Now I'm getting up and he's doing up his trousers. He's walking away and just looking back at me. He's climbing back over the wall. I can just hear his footsteps fading away as he was walking very fast. I'm kneeling there and crying.
33. I feel really guilty, disgusted and embarrassed, as though everyone would know what I'd done. I want to say something to my mum and dad, but felt it was my fault. I shouldn't have gone scrumping behind that wall – so I never said anything.
34. At the tea table that night mum asked me what I'd been doing that day, I was blushing and was very embarrassed – I felt she could tell just by looking at me. I tried to tell her I'd been playing in the park but I could hardly get the words out.
35. It seemed too awful to keep thinking about, I prayed it had never happened. Nobody knew – it was my guilty secret.

At this point I intervened and did some checking. I will just briefly mention that it has to do with making sure that there is not an interrelated repression lurking close to the surface.

Post-session conversation went roughly as follows:

Me: Well, Mr Client, I promised you a moment of 'surprising and liberating enlightenment'. How about it?

Him: Well, ten out of ten for 'surprising'. I would never have believed that – but I remember it so clearly now. Liberating? Yes, I certainly feel as though something inside of me has been lifted. Like a cloud lifted. Enlightenment? Well . . . I can think of one thing off the cuff – my friends have motorbikes and I'm still keen. They go down the woods at weekends – but I only went once. I was nearly sick under those trees. I know why now, don't I?

Me: Nothing else you've particularly noticed, then?

Him: Well, I certainly feel a sense of relief . . . and there's lots of things coming clear – particularly about my sex life. I'd often been frightened I was queer. What was it you had in mind particularly?

Me: You haven't noticed that you've stopped stuttering then?

Him: Oh boy! I'm not, am I. That must have started when my mum was cross-questioning me at the tea table. Do you think that's why I blush so much as well?

And that's that. Exit one convert to analysis. He will perhaps have the odd moment of anxiety and even difficulty with his words for the next day or two until he stops dissecting it, lets it all drift back where it belongs – back in his past. His intellect has seen it, and dealt with it, but now he knows – there just are not better words to describe the feeling than 'surprising and liberating enlightenment'.

Look at the thirty-five recollections of his that I have listed and see how each one has an indirect reference to the complex we were in search of. Look at the 'automatic writing' and compare it with the only words spoken during the assault.

We, and he, have the advantage of hindsight, which makes all things clear. But hindsight has to be acquired, it has to be achieved, and it has to be worked for; even more amazing, he will need hindsight to notice that his symptoms have in fact gone. He will only notice his fear of trees, his stutter and such have gone, as he looks back with the hindsight that he daily acquires. Ask yourself this: Did you wake up this morning and say, 'Oh good, I haven't got a toothache'?

The case I have used as an illustration was extremely straightforward, quick to conclude and devoid of any side-tracking complications, and the client's natural recalcitrance was easy to overcome. I hope by this stage you will not join the chorus of unenlightened and say: 'But surely he could have remembered that on his own'; 'He couldn't possibly have forgotten that'; 'I had something worse than that happen to me but I didn't forget'; 'Surely that couldn't have made him stutter' . . . . Mankind's reluctance to accept the principle of psychosomatic ailments hovers perilously close to megalomania of the species. 'Actually, it's quite all right for these things to be psychosomatic in other people, but not, of course, in me.'

MIGRAINE

Let us take as an example the blight of migraine, which has been studied for over 2000 years, though modern medicine is no nearer a solution than were the Romans. Its effects are felt by over 5 000 000 people in the UK alone. It has broken more marriages, ruined more chances of promotion and upset more plans than any other blight of man. Almost one in ten people suffer migraine attacks, and we have all seen the devastating effect on people's lives. Individual symptoms vary, but often include blinding headache, sickness and nausea, flashing light in vision, or disturbed or out-of-focus eyesight with a strong reaction to bright light.

One singularly unusual fact that came to light many years ago is that although it seems to be a blight upon the whole world, affecting every race, colour and creed, there is one notable exception: migraine is absolutely unknown in primitive African tribes.

At first glance that would lend credence to the belief that migraine is an illness of modern civilization, but, that being the case, why did the Romans suffer from it 2000 years ago? The conclusion reached was that, rather than it being something we are doing in our civilization which produces migraine, perhaps it is something we are *not* doing. Perhaps the primitive African tribes are doing something which renders migraine impossible. Diet was ruled out because none of the cases investigated (who had been Westernized after an African upbringing), had succumbed in any way to migraine. Likewise climate and weather conditions were discounted for the same reason. Yet diet, in particular, is the supposed cause upon which modern medicine firmly hangs its hat, and migraine sufferers are subjected to the further restrictions of no cheese, chocolate, etc. Indeed it can sometimes be shown that a particular foodstuff will precipitate an attack. Could it be that, yet again, medicine is treating only the effects and not the causes?

Think for a moment of those primitive African tribes, and the importance they attach to the transition from youth to maturity. The puberty initiation ceremonies for both boys and girls contain ritualistic procedures which have been handed down through time, and one of the basic themes is the symbolic casting out of the devil and evil spirits. The ritual dancing, the ceremony, the symbolic smoking and the monotonous chanting of these initiations have all the necessary elements to produce a light hypnotic trance in the participants – and a light, lethargic state of hypnosis is just about the 'bees-knees' when it comes to winkling out repressions. Surely it is blindingly obvious – it is to me – that the African tribes are immune to migraines because they dispel these repressions, these childhood anxieties, at the correct time – at the transition from youth to maturity, effectively banishing their symbolic evil spirits – in reality their hang-ups of youth.

'Lest you come to me as little children . . .' No! I promise not to bring religion into this, or add any fuel to the theory: Jesus Christ – hypnotist. I've read what poor old Sigmund heaped upon his shoulders when he tried to explain that particular hornets' nest.

The more you think about migraine simply being a 'blanketing action' of the mind, a shutting-out of consciousness of unpalatable memories and emotions, the more it makes sense. Supposing the stutterer I quoted with his 'man in the brown suit' had been a migraine sufferer. He would likely have got a migraine every time he went under trees, every time he saw a man dressed in a brown suit, every time he had sex. All those things would subconsciously have triggered an attempt at recall, which the mind prohibits – of course he would never have consciously seen the connections. Can you see why milk, cheese, chocolate, etc., are the arch-enemy of the migraine sufferer? Can you think of more likely foodstuffs to trigger subconscious recall of childhood?

What I am saying, of sheer necessity, implies that every human being is walking around stuffed full of repressions which could have been fairly easily released at the time of puberty. All right, I won't simply imply it – I'll say it. Every human being is walking around stuffed full of repressions which could have been fairly easily released at the time of puberty.

It takes only seconds for an incident or emotion to arise strong enough to succumb to repression and our childhood to puberty is made up of around four hundred million seconds.

I will go a step further. You are learning to do something that should never be necessary in the first place. There should never be any need for psychoanalysis; there should be no such things as phobias, psychosomatic bodily symptoms or people externalizing and identifying their anxieties.

CHILDREN

Give me a class of 11-12-year-olds. Let me induct them into hypnosis. Children are fantastic subjects, by the way; they love it and accept it without the stupid qualms and prejudices many adults express.) That classful of kids in hypnosis – let me take them through 'Session one' as I described it . . . the cathartic effect will take place without them needing to say a word. The discharge of the emotion will suffice and you will see some emotion in that classroom. That emotion would quickly pass, leaving them none the worse for their adventure. None the worse! Did I really say none the worse? Those kids will be the most rational, logical, straight-forward, uncomplicated, nice people you will ever meet in later life. Give me a world full of such people and I'll resign my cynicism tomorrow.

They, as adults, would insist on their children going through such an experience. Oops! Just as my fantasy was going so nicely . . . before I could do all this I'd have to get their parents' permission though, wouldn't I? . . . and the schoolteachers . . . and the education authority . . . and perhaps even Parliament. Still – shouldn't be difficult . . . surely they'll understand when I explain . . . won't they? Ah well, it was a nice fantasy for a moment.

I believe that such a process should be possible, should be allowed, nay, encouraged and that the effects within a decade would be to reduce the costs of the National Health Service enormously. I cannot see the manufacturers of diazepam (Valium) being too pleased though. John Lennon sang, 'You may call me a dreamer, but I'm not the only one' in his song 'Imagine'. Well, I do not want to be the only one either.

8. TRANSFERENCE AND RESISTANCE

Now I am going to try and explain the phenomenon of transference, because until you fully understand it you will never wholly realize why the client could not get to his own repressions without you to help him. Even as I begin, I have already floundered by inferring you will ever come fully to understand transference. I would claim to know more than a fair amount about the phenomenon – and yet I know I do not fully understand it.

Transference has been variously described by numerous writers, and that in itself is unusual. Medical men do not feel the need to write about how their patients respect them, look up to them, appreciate their 'bedside manner', accept their assurances that they will be better in a few days, accept that the medicine will do them good, and so on; and yet these things are every bit as deserving of the title 'transference'.

We are not only going to discuss, dissect, evaluate and generally question transference, but at a given point at the end of our analysis we are going to do our level best to make our client dissolve it, get rid of it, revert back to being totally indifferent to us, as he was before he commenced analysis. Should we not be able to bring him to that indifference again, then we have not cured him, he has fallen into the grip of the 'transference neurosis'. He is just as ill of transference as ever he was of migraine, or stutters, or twitches, or anxiety, or whatever. Only when the transference has finally been cleared away does the person come to full internal insight and enlightenment; only then do all his symptoms disappear.

Herein lies the fundamental difference between analysis and any other form of therapy. We aim to bring about an internal change in the person, and that internal change does not want to be as a result of anything we said. 'I will give you one piece of advice, and one piece only, and that is to take nobody's advice – and that includes the advice I have just given you.'

In a doctor–patient relationship it is good that the patient retains transference. Let's face it, the most marvellous medication available would stand little chance if your doctor said, 'Well, you can take it if you like, but I think it useless.' On the other hand, if he gave you a sugar-coated salt tablet and assured you it would cure your headache, then the placebo effect would probably ensure the disappearance of your headache. We would not be dealing with analysis if we did not appreciate that we were dealing with subconscious forces. Subconscious forces create transference, and only by its dissolution can we be assured that the forces are no longer at work.

The textbooks call transference a strange mixture of hostility, suspicion, affection and jealousy; a tendency to react to the analyst in ways in which the subject reacted to other important figures in his life. Words cannot do it justice. Remember earlier I said we humans used our process of recall in seven forms: incident only, incident plus emotion, emotion only, etc. Hypnosis aids particularly the recall of emotion, so as a person dutifully recounts incidents from his past he is going to feel little twinges of emotion and sometimes the emotion only, with no recall to accompany it. In the Enchiridion, the philosopher Epictetus was at pains to point out that men are not influenced by events, but only by their interpretation of those events. Ellis, Brandt, and other great men of today, have elaborated this theory to create the *Therapies of Rational Behaviour*, and *Rational Self-counselling*. I would not presume to summarize their writings, but only to borrow from them as Dr Brandt's explanation of emotions is a good one. He says our emotions are made up of perceptions, thoughts, and then emotive feelings. In other words, you perceive the event, you think about it or 'tell yourself' something about it, and then, and then only, do you experience the emotive feeling.

When an emotion wells up, like a bubble surfacing, as a result of the hypnotic experience and the process of recall, the intellect is left floundering. What happens next is very similar to the process which takes place in the development of a phobia, when the person has to rationalize his anxiety. He is experiencing an emotion, the anxiety, for no known reason. So, he gets to know one – he projects his anxiety onto the phobic object or situation in the environment. Well, in analysis a very similar things happens. The client experiences an emotion and projects it outwards. Guess where! Well, he has his eyes closed so there are not many situations in the environment or objects he can light upon. As far as he is concerned there is only one thing of any importance anywhere near: *the analyst*. He will feel the surfacing emotion for the analyst, thereafter his relationship with the analyst will be tinged by that emotion until a fresh one comes along – not to replace it, but to add to it. No wonder transference is such a strange mixture of hostility, suspicion, affection, jealousy and so on.

These emotions have been bottled up a long time, and they are strong emotions. Oh boy, are they strong emotions! There is nobody who can hate, love, suspect and so on, as can a client in analysis. How does he cope with it? How in fact does the analyst cope with it? Well, I feel like fatuously saying, 'with great difficulty'. But that will not suffice. It has got to be lived through by the client; it has got to be experienced . . . and don't sit there smugly thinking the analyst is immune. If, after all my words to date, you still think that none of all this applies to you, then for goodness sake go to the pub and don't waste your time reading any more.

The analyst 'appreciates the good fortune which has enabled him to give his assistance to such a particularly valuable personality'. Not every time, surely? Yes, every time. But surely some of your clients are paranoids? I still say, every time. But surely some of your clients aren't nice people? I still say, every time . . . and stop calling me Shirley!

The client starts to take an unusual interest in the analyst. He is fascinated by him, tends to over-value his qualities and bores everyone about how clever and wonderful his shrink is – that is, unless the transference has taken on an erotic tinge, in which case he usually, but not always, goes quiet about it (particularly if it is a male client and male analyst). Bit by bit, emotion by emotion, the analyst is changing in the eyes and mind of the client. In fact, subconsciously, the analyst is becoming somebody else, somebody from the client's past, sometimes only an imaginary person from the person's past.

One thing you must appreciate about transference is that it is neurotic – in the true sense of the word. It is created from a neurosis so must inevitably be itself neurotic, and in consequence does not take any account of normality, or that which is considered normal. Thus, if the analyst is male, seventy and ugly, he is still likely to observe his client (say, female, eighteen and beautiful) falling into the grip of an erotic fascination for him; or, if the analyst is female and thirty, she is still likely to observe her female client (of, say, fifty) beginning to treat her as though she was the client's mother. Transference being spawned by juvenile emotions, is itself a childish, or 'rather' juvenile, thing; and just as the juvenile finds it difficult to conceal his emotions and feelings, so too, the client in transference finds it difficult, indeed, quite often doesn't want, to conceal his feelings. Guilt wants to feel guilty; desire wants to feel desire; hate wants to feel hate, and so on.

Just as there is no such thing as a hypnotized feeling – no way of knowing you're in hypnosis, for reasons which I hope by now you have grasped; namely, we do not know our subconscious and so cannot ascribe our feelings to it, we rationalize them instead – so too, there is no way of knowing that your feelings are transference. Feelings are feelings, emotions are emotions, and if the client suddenly feels the overwhelming desire just to be with the analyst, just to look at him, and talk to him, then it will take a lot of self-control on his part not to give in to that desire.

I said that, in analysis, we were going to bring about an internal change in the person, and although I have asked you to try and absorb these writings without criticism, I should be most surprised if the thought did not, at the time, flicker through your mind that people cannot be changed; that, in any case, they are predisposed to behave the way they do. I hope the thought did flicker through your mind, because at least it shows you appreciate the enormity of what we attempt. Let me borrow Sigmund Freud's words yet again, when he said that 'the neurotic who is cured has really become another man, though at bottom, of course, he has remained the same'. I think what dear Sigis was trying to get across was that the person was destined to become the best person he could be, except for the cruel intervention of fate, which then intruded. We help the person remove that intervention of fate, we release him from his time warp, and he now develops naturally and freely into the best person he could be. Before analysis he was held in the vice-like grip of his neurosis, literally in a time warp. He was like a child, but desperately concealing that fact. For a while in analysis he will not even try and conceal that fact, at least not with the analyst, and will behave like a precocious child or turbulent teenager in revolt, or whatever his transference dictates at the time.

With regular inevitability the transference will take an erotic turn. What then, when the lady client, who has a male analyst, is thinking to herself, 'My goodness, if he only knew what was going through my mind at the moment.' The fact that she has pledged to say whatever comes into her mind conveniently escapes her memory at that moment. She fights a battle with herself. A purely conscious struggle with her emotions. This struggle has taken place once before, and last time she lost . . . or she won . . . whichever way you view it. Last time round the emotion was too much; the conflict was too great for the then still maturing mind, and the feelings, emotions, and possibly the incident, succumbed to repression. Now they are out again, the same emotions and feelings, fighting in the open – well, nearly in the open – but transferred to the analyst. To win or lose now does not matter a hang; it is all just a conscious conflict. The incident cannot possibly succumb to repression again; the person it too mature.

The feelings, though, can be jumped on. No, no, I don't mean any puns. I mean the person can find herself objecting most strongly to the feelings that she is getting, and vowing not to feel them any more; that she is going for treatment to get better, not to find 'that sort of feeling' interfering with the treatment. Next week she arrives, like Miss Goody Two Shoes, all prim and proper, and in a high state of resistance. In putting down her feelings so strongly, she has put down the very process which is carrying the analysis forward. A good analyst should have viewed all this unspoken body language with a good-humoured tolerance and then said something like: 'You seem a bit different somehow this week. We seemed to be getting on like a house on fire last week, and now you've gone all distant on me. Has someone upset you, or is it me?'

Wow! Talk about taking the bull by the horns, and she thought she had concealed it all so well. If necessary I would go a bit further: 'I did mention I wanted you to disclose all your thoughts and emotions, didn't I? I mean, I can see if you are crying, but I wouldn't be able to see if you were sexually aroused, would I?' If necessary, I'd go a bit further: 'I'm sorry, I'm making you blush, I guess you must have been feeling a bit excited over something last week, then?' One writer called it 'shaking the tree of transference' when you 'gently hint' that the person might have been thinking about the analyst during the week. Gentle hint, nothing! We have not gone to all the trouble of reviving this conflict to have her prissie, psuedo mid-Victorian morality interfere with the process. That is one of the things that is wrong with her anyway, so you can be sure we will definitely be bringing about an internal change in her morality.

The phenomenon of transference and phenomenon of resistance are intertwined. Of the two, resistance is surely the more understandable; after all, if there was not an internal resistance to finding out the contents of the repressed material, then it would never have been repressed in the first place. That of course is not the way your client sees it, and your client would say, 'I'm not resisting. I want to know what it is. I want to get better.' But common sense tells you that there must be a major subconscious resistance taking place, or he would do just as he intellectually says he wants to do and recall the repressed incident. Grasp here and now that you cannot release your own repressions, only other people's, because the vehicle of release is transference and if you are a compassionate person, look back with different eyes at the man I have mentioned so much, Sigmund Freud, and realize the sadness of fate which dictated that he keep his own neuroses to the grave, not in the same way as others do, who, forgive them, know not what they do, but knowingly. His own 'externalization and identification' must have been near total.

When I say that transference and resistance are intertwined, I use the word 'intertwined' as meaning 'most complexly woven together'. Transference breaks down resistance, but transference also creates resistance. Resistance creates transference, but resistance also breaks down transference. How about that for intertwined?

Think back to what I said about the client in session five, when the repression starts releasing, and he 'sees' something, as though on film. The resistance usually takes over very strongly then, as the intellect tries to dismiss it all as imagination. The transference keeps him at it. He wants to please you. The only way he can totally please you is to release the repression. Like a naughty child – own up. So he has got to keep at it. The resistance makes him want to stop, perhaps using the transference. So the lady client declares her love and desire. The fact that she's only known you for four hours, that you're twenty years younger, or twenty years older than her, that she knows you're married, etc., etc. – none of these things matter. The transference is a neurosis of equal strength to the neurosis that was brought for treatment. She loves you with the intensity of youth, even though she is perhaps sixty plus. Now she has declared it again. Like the child, however, that won't do . . . that's not enough . . . the transference demands more. The young fellow in analysis finds himself reacting to the mature male analyst as a parental figure – originally that lad had wanted to be as good as his own dad, then he wanted to be better than him, and that same conflict is re-created with the analyst. The resistance subconsciously tells him to stop the session, declaring there is nothing to be found – that way both resistance and transference are satisfied. The transference gets its own way by 'winning' over the parental figure, who 'loses' as being wrong. The resistance triumphs by stopping the session. Probably all of that would just be thought out as a conscious conflict, with the client lying there thinking, 'Any minute now I'll tell him this is all nonsense and getting us nowhere.' Should the resistance and transference entwine – so that it actually happens, so he stops the session – then the only salvation is explanation. For this and similar purposes, I keep Freud's writings in paperback in my consulting room, with various passages underlined in ink. I would just throw the book on my desk open at the relevant passage: 'Sometimes one gets an impression the person has replaced his intention of making an end to the problem by the alternative one of putting the analyst in the wrong and of triumphing over him.' When the lad has read it, he would likely say, 'Do you think I'm really doing that. Is that me?' I would probably not even answer, other than saying, 'Would you care to get back on the couch and we'll proceed' – or something after that style.

I have barely scratched the surface of transference and resistance, but already I hope you can see that analysis bears no resemblance to going to your doctor and asking for something to calm you down a bit. The most complex of forces are now at work and only about one in thirty clients would proceed through analysis as easily and comparatively uneventfully as the stutterer I discussed earlier.

Without doubt the hardest client ever for you to deal with is the person you know personally before analysis. Should it be necessary for you to continue knowing them post-analysis, then as a rule of thumb – don't. Don't know them before analysis, don't take them into analysis if you know them, don't know them after analysis. Life, of course, is made up of don't and can'ts, and mustn'ts and shouldn'ts, and here of course is one of those intangibles I said you would always be stuck with if you involved yourself with the human psyche and its failings: at least if you do one of the don'ts you will know what you are doing.

SYMPTOMS – AFFECTED BY TRANSFERENCE

People have only two forms of symptoms: they are either direct symptoms or indirect symptoms. The direct symptoms are directly as a result of the internal conflict taking place in the person. The indirect symptoms, you will not be surprised to hear, are indirectly as a result of the internal conflict within the person.

Back for a moment to that stutterer we discussed in Chapter 7. Direct symptoms (that we know of): predisposed to blush – because of subconscious guilt; fear of homosexuality – because of repressed happening; anxiety – because of the actual internal conflict. Indirect symptoms: nail-biting – because of the anxiety; smoking – because of the anxiety; dendrophobia (fear of trees) – because of the anxiety; and, of course, the stuttering itself – again because of the anxiety.

From a practical point of view there is an amazing difference between the forms: the direct symptoms will disappear as the original conflict is exposed and released – actually at the moment of the release, the catharsis, if you like. The direct symptoms will then go, and go for ever. The indirect symptoms will not yet disappear, although much of the intensity will go from them. The indirect symptoms are caught up in the transference and will not go until the transference is gone. Should the transference last five years, then the symptoms will survive five years. They will go only when transference goes. Understand now why I said 'Don't' a few times before, but also realize this: you cannot dissolve transference for the person; he has got to do that himself. You can help, but you cannot actually do it for him – and he will often resist dissolving transference every bit as strongly as he resisted finding the unconscious causes of his anxiety. Not only that, he has no way of knowing that he is in the grip of transference and not just a 'normal' emotion, because of course the transference is a normal emotion, albeit neurotically created.

Any clearer yet? Or have I just totally confused you? I suspect from the foregoing you might be puzzled about the stuttering fellow I described – on the face of it he demonstrated nothing of what I now describe. Well, two points: I did say he represented only one in thirty clients and the case was uncomplicated; secondly, he does, unknowingly, and not very apparently, demonstrate what I am now talking about. His resistance? Well, he took a lot of persuasion actually to start his motor up and start dishing out the recollections. He mentioned in the last session that he might have to stop the session soon, he was getting so anxious. It turns out he was resisting, but not very much. Transference? Well, here was a shy sort of fellow, somewhat self-deprecating, predisposed to blushing, in fact a bit of an inferiority complex case. How did he deal with me? In a word 'respectfully', as he had dealt with other major figures in his life. He did as he was told. He would not say 'boo' to a goose, and that's exactly the form the transference took with me. His relief at the repressed recollection was so great he dissolved transference practically there and then. However, you can bet that, between sessions, he, who was to say afterwards he'd always been worried about his sexual inclinations, had entertained the odd fantasy about me. The 'rules' of analysis require him to disclose such thoughts, but 't'would be a braver man than he, Gungha Dhin'. All of that he saw quite clearly with his moment of enlightenment, so transference was doomed there and then.

Just to throw another little spanner in the workings before I move on. Consider this: the person does not know that his feelings and emotions from subconscious and conscious forces joining are transference. His direct symptoms have gone, his indirect symptoms have toned down, lost their intensity, and, as previously stated, nobody could possibly have any conception of what he would be like if he was different. He can see no reason to dissolve transference, indeed, does not know how to dissolve transference even if he did want to. What happens, of course, is that the transference does work its course until the sheer impossibility of it finally dictates its demise.

Now I want to explain the unexplainable again, so please bear with me some more. Why do the indirect symptoms survive until the dissolution of transference? That is the unexplainable I want to explain.

When a repressed memory surfaces, the intellect, which knows nothing of the incident or complex, attempts to deny the veracity of it all, and would prefer to dismiss it as imagination. The emotions make this rather difficult of course – it is one thing to imagine an emotion, say fear, for example, but it is quite another matter to feel the fear – that is real. At first the client is telling you something which his intellect is attempting to dismiss as imagination. He is compelled towards a belief in the reality of the incident by two principal factors: one, that he is experiencing emotions which match the incident; and the other, that you had prophesied all this would take place, and he is in the grip of transference to you. Only when the transference is finally dissolved does the person come to a sense of inner conviction – it could hardly be anything to do with you then, because effectively you do not exist any more. There you are, I managed to explain it quite easily, except that it is not really as simple as I have portrayed it – there are other interwoven factors at work.

Somewhat earlier I glibly said there were many reasons why analysis has never caught on as an 'in' therapy, and transference and resistance form well over 50 per cent of the reasons. The analyst at the receiving end (and to some extent the sharp end) of transference and resistance has to have a very unusual personality, and if I now sound somewhat self-deprecating perhaps it will compensate for some of my earlier apparent conceit. I chose the word 'unusual' quite deliberately, out of many others which might seem far more appropriate. Others would perhaps prefer adjectives such as: strong, moral, honest, professional, plausible, empathic, resilient, to name but a few. I'll stick with 'unusual' and don't propose to elaborate further. Here I will leave you to draw your own conclusions, be they right or wrong, from what you have understood so far.

Another of the objections to analysis is, of course, the sheer unbelievable aspects of it. Perhaps it is somewhat remiss of me to have used such a simplified example as our ex-stuttering friend, and perhaps I ought to have tried to guide you through the more complex structures of a far more typical client. Now, I pledge, here and now, that the man in the brown suit is real, he existed, the client occurred as I have described; I have taken no poetic licence at all – the case notes still exist in my records – but I make no apologies for having quite deliberately chosen for illustration a case that is very easy to follow.

THE SUBCONSCIOUS DICTATING WHAT WE SAY

We do not necessarily say what we are thinking. We do not necessarily express that which is on our minds, be it conscious or subconscious. The term 'Freudian slip' did not become popular without reason. Let us look at the illustration of you having forgotten a person's name. As you struggle to remember, you find names presenting themselves to your mind . . . Turpin . . . Rounder . . . Woodman . . . Better . . . Lana . . . Suddenly, you give up, you relax, you turn round, and as you turn round, the name springs to your mind – Turner. That's it, Turner.

Line them up:

Turpin ....Turner
Rounder ....Turner
Woodman ....Turner (wood turner)
Better ....Turner
Lana ....Turner (Lana Turner)

The name Turner must have been hovering very close to the surface or the other names could not have presented themselves. It is no coincidence that our ex-stutterer told us how he remembered 'running around the hedges in the back garden which his father had cut in the shape of birds'. Subconsciously he must have had the incident which took place under the other trees on his mind.

Imagine now a client in analysis producing the following sequence of memories:

1. I remember my brother stealing my money.
2. I remember getting caned on the hand for fighting at school.
3. I remember my brother going into hospital after breaking his leg.
4. I remember burning my hand on a hot iron.
5. I remember being jealous of my brother and wishing him harm.
6. I remember cutting my hand with a knife.

In that imaginary sequence, I would be expecting the imaginary client to release a repressed memory of attacking his brother with a knife – I might be wrong, but that is what I would be expecting.

Look at the sequence of recollections again and see if you can understand why I think that they would release that particular repression. Now look at the following sequence:

1 I remember lying in bed on a Sunday morning.
2 I remember getting caned on my hands.
3 I remember taking ages in the bathroom.
4 I remember picking up a red-hot dish.
5 I often used to lock myself in the toilet.
6 I once got caught for stealing – I got caned for that too.
7 I had a wet dream once.
8 I was told sex was dirty.

If you are not expecting masturbation guilt to be released very soon, then I have been wasting my breath – sorry – ink! You must be able to see that by now; if you honestly cannot, give up – if you really cannot see that now then you would not make an analyst and you will never truly understand hypnosis. Sit in judgement upon yourself now because if you have really understood that which I have so far written, then soon I must, of sheer necessity, start to become a bit of a bore, by labouring points which are so obvious to you, that you wonder why I keep labouring them. If you haven't understood, then please, please go back – go back to page one. Read again. The enlightenment is there for the taking, and our jigsaw should be making the beginnings of a very clear picture.

Assuming that you are still reading on, or that you have waded right the way through again, and have reached this point once more, take this on board as well: consciously saying something, close to, and indirectly related to, what we are subconsciously thinking, is not of course confined to the analyst's couch. If you have really grasped what I have told you, and not only think you have grasped it, then in future your friends and acquaintances can have few secrets from you. You will often realize what they are subconsciously thinking by what they are saying, even if they do not consciously realize it themselves. After a few instances of you answering, accidentally, their subconscious – the unspoken thought which had prompted the conscious words, you may well find your perception losing you friends. The world may well be a stage, and we may well be the actors and actresses, but we are none too keen on anyone seeing through our make-up and showbiz garb, to the sometimes rather shallow character underneath.

Without a doubt the most difficult part of analysis is the easiest part. Yet another contradiction in terms, but nonetheless true. To get to the repressions the analysis uses the most trivial of recollections and, although these are very easy for the person to produce, it is difficult to get him to voice these recollections. Disregarding the obvious difficulties – such as the 'fact' that such a trivial recollection, which was already within the conscious recall of the client, appears, to him, to be totally irrelevant to the whole proceedings and therefore of no account and not worth repeating – as well as other difficulties, realize also that the client feels very silly. Certainly in the opening sessions, the person feels silly. To be sure, the state of lethargic hypnosis part-way overcomes his vague feelings of embarrassment at reciting such trivial thoughts, but for all that, he still feels silly. You will need to exercise a lot of 'personality', at session two in particular, in order to get the wheels rolling.

I think while I am mentioning difficulties I will touch on another one: the 'erroneous association'. Let me use an illustration to explain firstly what we mean by the term erroneous association. A man in his mid-thirties consults with 'physical impotence'. He explains that whenever the time comes actually to have sex with a girl, his penis limply subsides, making intercourse impossible. However, he 'knows' what caused it all and wants you just to use hypnosis to 'blank out' the cause from his mind, then he knows he will be cured. He elaborates upon the cause as dating from the very first time he ever got the opportunity to have sex. He was in the army, aged eighteen, and it was a brothel in Singapore. Unfortunately the girl in question smelled rather offensively, and this put him off at the last minute so that he lost his erection and couldn't proceed. She had laughed at him and called him a 'cherry boy'. He further explained that the next time he got a chance to go with a girl he found the words 'cherry boy' almost ringing in his ears, and could practically smell that first girl all over again – this 'of course' was the reason why he failed so dismally that second time. From then on it had been similar most times, with just the odd success through the years . . . Now that is an erroneous association. He believes he knows the cause of his problem, having wrongly associated it with that first misadventure.

When I mentioned 'erroneous association' as a difficulty, I was not really thinking of the difficulty of convincing him that, far from blanking out memories of the past, we are going to dredge up ones that he does not even know about. With that particular difficulty he is no different – no easier, no harder – than the rest of a doubting humanity. I was thinking of the technical difficulty in analysis, when the erroneous association keeps popping up with the annoying regularity so he says, 'My mind has gone again to the brothel in Singapore.' What he really means is 'My intellect has just intruded and said I know what caused my problem so there is no point in continuing this search amongst my other recollections'. What do you do? Why, you keep your patience and you say, 'Fine, again just let you thoughts drift and tell me the very next thing that you find yourself thinking of.' Did I mention somewhere along the line, that in that 'unusual' personality of the analyst there has to be an in-built patience, because quite often in analysis, rather as in the mating of elephants, there is a lot of huffing, there is a lot of puffing, but then nothing happens for an awfully long time.

As I start to meander down these difficult roads, to talk of transference, resistance, complications and problems, I want to try and avoid making it all sound impossible – because it is not. Yet I want to forewarn and forearm you to the various ramifications. Einstein asserted his theory of relativity, and it does not just relate to space and time, it relates to all things. There is no such thing as an unsuccessful analysis, but that does not mean to say that every analysis will proceed to a successful conclusion, and once again this apparent disputation, so seemingly self-refutatory, is true. Should a person experience session one, and session one alone, and then never return – that person has come to a greater insight of himself than before; he is improved as a person.

I am reminded of the chap who rang to say that twelve months after he had seen me for a suggestion therapy to combat smoking, he had foolishly started smoking again, and would like to return for a further session, in order to stop again. I joked with him on the phone and laughed that it was all good for the trade and that his silliness would cost him my session fees. His reply was to the effect that if my fee was £5000 it would still have been worth it. He went on to explain that, in the session, I had asked him to let his mind drift back into his younger years for the source of upset which was strong enough to make him smoke in later life. (I very seldom do that in suggestion therapy sessions, by the way, because it can have the effect of making the person rather anxious and uptight for the next few days, thereby increasing their desire to smoke, nail-bite, or whatever.) He further explained that, prior to that session, he had suffered migraines at the rate of at least three a week for at least twenty years, and that subsequent to the therapy, he had not had a single attack of migraine. When he presented himself for the anti-smoking session I asked him if he minded disclosing what he had recalled, and he elaborated that he had been horrified to find himself recalling masturbating as a teenager to a fantasy of his own mother. He was an intelligent man, and he was able to realize that the recollection had been concealed from his normal intellectual awareness, and he could clearly recall that he had experienced an emotion of intense shame as the memory returned to him in the session.

A classic example of the awesome potential of the hypnotic state. Significantly, though, as if to prove everything I have told you, he had not felt the need to ring me up and thank me. He had not felt the need to announce to a waiting world that there is a cure for migraine. He certainly had not felt the need to send me the £5000 he said it was worth. Had it not been for the intrusion of fate, sending him back to the filthy weed, I would never have known of the cure. But there again . . . perhaps he was subconsciously driven to . . . smoke again . . . in order to return to me . . . in order to tell me of the internal change. I certainly wouldn't bet against it – would you? Cause and effect.

REJECTION BY THE ESTABLISHMENT

Hipolyte Bernheim (1837–1919), who practised with Liebault at the Nancy School of Hypnotism, pointed out that many people are horrified by anything apparently amazing – they will deny facts because those facts do not agree with the established conceptions in their minds. He added that facts are facts, and as such are undeniable, and if the interpretation is faulty, not to blame the facts, but rather blame the insufficiency of the person's knowledge . . .

Carl Gustav Jung in June 1928 accurately, without at that time realizing it, forecast the possibility of the inhuman horrors of World War II (or III, for that matter) in his criticism of large organizations. He made the point that here was piled up and accentuated man, and of course, all that is primitive in man – the person's individuality submerged in the interests of the great monstrosity that each organization is. He added, what we can, and have observed, that the greatest infamy on the part of the organization will not disturb the individual, so long as the majority resolutely believe in the righteousness of their cause . . ..

I have reason for quoting the above two great men, for I want to free the cures brought about by analysis 'under' hypnosis, from the slightest suspicion of being cures of suggestion, and at the same time hopefully to convince you, if you are an open-minded person of reason, that the truths of analysis are indeed truths and their non-acceptance by 'great organizations' is as explainable, as understandable, as their rejection by an individual. British psychiatry is largely, and not surprisingly, controlled by British psychiatrists, heavily entrenched in the status quo – the medical profession assuredly justifies the title of 'large organization'.

Freud, and his brainchild psychoanalysis, have endured every criticism one could countenance, and it is considered common knowledge that Freud was supposedly shattered to discover that reports, in analysis, from adult patients of 'seduction' in their infant years, had been 'proved' false by other members of the family who asserted such sexual happenings never took place.

Bear with me – the last four apparently disjointed paragraphs are leading me somewhere.

Firstly, Freud talked to his clients too much (and this from me, who hardly ever uses one word when ten will do). The less you say to a client once the process has commenced the better. Your knowledge and awareness, your theories and perception – they are nothing to the client. You do not, and should not, expound your interpretation to the person. From the outset you should always try to avoid giving any direction to the analysis at all.

Secondly, the misinformed – 'resolutely believing in the righteousness of their cause' having read, for instance, the Oedipus complex, as outlined by Freud – have assumed (with their 'normal' thinking) that Freud inferred we were aware of those matters, and that discussion could elicit the same. Well, I cannot think of any single thing more designed to alienate a client than to start discussing with him the fact that in his early development he had incestuous designs upon his mother. Notice here I use the word 'fact' – and before you do a Hipolyte Bernheim on me and reject the fact with horror, because of the insufficiency of your knowledge, look back to where I described the Oedipus complex in Chapter 4, when I was talking about the split-off between affection and eroticism in our sexuality.

Modern psychiatry rejects these and other explanations of infantile sexuality, from the same insufficiency of knowledge. Being a 'large organization' they can complacently reject the odd little individual doubt from the individual within the organization, his individuality being sacrificed to the organization as a whole. Any of their ranks, who view electroconvulsive therapy (ECT), for example, with the same deprecating eye that I would use, considering it to be hovering upon the medieval, and somewhat barbaric, would find, of course, they could continue undisturbed with such infamy, knowing that the majority believed in the righteousness of their cause. It is perhaps interesting to mention that the only evidence which has ever been put forward to justify the electrical creation of an epileptic fit in a person's brain, is esoteric evidence; and as to why they ever tried it in the first place, nobody has yet explained. There again, the same can be said of the drug aspirin, so perhaps my criticism is not too valid.

All that which I have written and herein told you is true. Aristotle defined truth as follows: 'To say of what is, that it is not, or of what is not, that it is, is false. To say of what is, that it is, or of what is not, that it is not, is true.' Tarski said, 'A statement is true, if and only if, it corresponds to the facts.' Freud's undoing, together with others who have stumbled upon the truths of the subconscious, and the truths of analysis, and possibly my undoing now, is the sheer impossibility of tendering scientifically demonstrable facts to support such truths.

Analysis concerns that which is most intimate in a person's life. After analysis a person goes into a semi-disavowal state, e.g. 'I don't think I was ever that bad that I really needed to go to an analyst anyway.' We humans know that Claude Levi-Strauss hit a tremendous truth when he wrote: 'There is an "it" which thinks in me and makes me doubt whether it is I that think . . .'. Here is another truth: It is not possible to bring any person to harm with analysis under hypnosis. Can, the same, I wonder, be said of ECT, Valium, barbiturates, tranquillizers, surgical interventions and the like.

Understand now that the preceding pages of these writings are so much waste paper as far as a client is concerned. Your knowledge, your theories, are but droplets upon an ocean of controversy – again, as far as your client is concerned. Analysis does not thrust its theories down the client's throat. Its theories are not even mentioned, unless to contribute to the work in hand. The person must bring himself – using the analyst only as a catalyst – to an intellectual and emotional insight into his problem, so that he (not the analyst) understands the cause of his problem; so that he understands the origin of his problem, and so that he understands the true nature of his problem. With that insight and understanding, and with the discharge of emotion that takes place, an internal change takes place in the person.

I suspect that most people (psychiatrists included) imagine that the analyst waits only for the client to mention his father for the first time, and then pounces upon the poor client and elaborates for hours on end about his poor relationship with his father, his ambitions and so on – explaining to the client that of course this is what has caused his problems in life. Balderdash! The good analyst says very little once the analysis is well under way, confining himself perhaps to the occasional: 'That's fine, I want you to connect that last recollection in your thoughts with something else, and then tell me the very next thing you find yourself thinking about.' You could hardly be accused of inflicting your theories upon him, could you?

Probably the hardest part of being a good analyst is the fact that you will normally come to an awareness of the subconscious 'bug' your client needs to grub out, long before he does.

Go back for a moment to Chapter 7 and my illustrating case of the stutterer with his man in a brown suit. When the client mentioned the 'white wall' a couple of times and then also mentioned so apparently randomly and casually the 'man in the brown suit', I immediately put two and two together and, as it transpired, got the sum right. My intuition, based on a lot of experience, told me that it would not be long before he was releasing a repression to do with that man. But, suppose I had said to the client, 'I think that man in the brown suit probably did something to you' . . . Later, remember, the client got an apparent imaginary impression in his thoughts, consisting of the man climbing over the wall, approaching him and undoing his trousers. Bit by bit the recollection became real to him as his emotions finally convinced his ego, his intellect, to stand down, and release the memory.

> 'I did this,' says my memory.
>
> 'I cannot have done this,' says my pride . . . and remains inexorable.
>
> In the end – memory yields.

Now add a postscript: 'Pride surrenders to analyst and memory triumphs again.' What chance do you think that factual recollection would have stood of getting through if I had said such a silly thing as above? At the apparent imaginary stage of the recall the client would have said, 'I wish you hadn't said that about that man. You've gone and put it in my mind now – I can imagine him climbing over that wall after me.'

Moral? You do not make any such comment. Any suggestions you give are purely to encourage recall, and random recall at that. Are you beginning to see why I can be so categoric about our cures being internal changes and not the result of suggestion?

GREY AREAS

When we were infants, things at first were either symbolically black or white; with our growing perception we gradually became aware that there were infinite tones of grey in-between. Now I propose to splash enough grey around to paint a class 'F' destroyer.

Read the following extract from a client's recall and see if you spot the grey area.

1. I am remembering walking in the park with Mum and Dad and my brother.
2. Me and my brother lagged behind Mum and Dad to play by a shallow pond.
3. My brother threw my cap in the middle of the water and ran off.
4. That's funny, I don't actually remember this, it's almost like looking at it on film. I can see myself walking into the pond to get my cap.
5. I'm imagining that the bottom of the pond feels very, very muddy under my feet.
6. I could feel myself sinking into the mud – this is beginning to upset me. It feels very real – I can practically feel that mud now.
7. I can feel myself sinking deeper and deeper in the mud. I'm screaming but my parents don't hear. I feel absolutely terrified now, as I'm telling you, it's as real as if it was happening.

8. I can physically feel myself sinking right under the mud. It closes over the top of my head. I can see bubbles coming to the top of the surface of the mud as I just slowly sink under. I fear I'm dying. I know I'm dying. It's horrible, I'm going to open my eyes. I can't stand it – it's too awful.
9. I'm sorry I just had to open my eyes and stop. That was too awful. No wonder I've been claustrophobic all my life – and yet somehow that doesn't feel real. The feelings were very real, but somehow it's more like a dream – as though I'd make it up. It doesn't feel real.

Well, Sherlock, did you spot the pink/grey elephant? Elementary, my dear Watson – he couldn't have seen bubbles rising to the surface of the mud if he was under it, now could he? No! He's seen the same Tarzan movie you and I both saw, when we were kids, where the creature sank under the swamp in the green slime and bubbles appeared as it disappeared. You remember it, don't you?

What really happened? Be patient – patience is a virtue remember.

Next session: 'I've been thinking all week. I've decided that was imagination last week. I obviously just imagined it. Probably to please you.' You neither agree nor disagree. You do not inflict your opinion upon him. You will not even be drawn into discussion upon it. You just get the session under way as soon as possible. Just a cursory induction and then you shut up. After several random memories taking up about a third of the session, our client will likely proceed as follows:

10. I've gone back to thinking of that park again. Actually it's been at the back of my thoughts all the time I've been talking today.
11. I can see myself walking into that pond again to get my cap back. My brother's laughing at me as he runs off. There are two girls there laughing as well.
12. I walked into the pond. It was very muddy on the bottom. One of my shoes has come off. (Note the intermix of past and present.) I'm stuck in the mud trying to find my shoe. My cap is still a way off – I'm sinking in the mud.

13. I can definitely remember that. I lost my shoe. I'm sinking in the mud. I was terrified. It's a horrible feeling. I could imagine it eventually being in my mouth and eyes. I was terrified. I was screaming for Mum and Dad to come back. Oh Christ! . . . (Silence.)

'Go on, keep going, tell me the next thing that happened.'

14. I can't . . . I can't . . . Oh Christ . . . it's real, I know it's real, I remember now. God, I felt so ashamed. Those girls were laughing out loud. Mum and Dad came back. I tried to pretend it was mud running down my legs. I feel so dirty and ashamed now. I messed myself.
15. Do you know, that explains an awful lot. I've always gone to the toilet before I've gone out, even if I didn't want to go, and I've insisted on my kids doing the same. Oh! And . . . (etc., etc.)

Once again, mark it 'Repression released, case closed'. It was not such a grey area after all, was it? The waters are just a bit muddier to see through occasionally.

Here is another example, taken from the notes of a lady client.

1. I can 'see' in my thoughts a picture, like a film, of my dad breaking my bedroom door down and me cowering away from him. I'm lying on the bed.
2. I can 'see' in my thoughts a picture of the milkman looking in through my bedroom window. I'm lying on my bed again. This doesn't make sense.
3. This is daft. I can 'see' in my thoughts my brother. He's peeping through the keyhole into my bedroom. I'm lying on my bed again. There wasn't a keyhole in my door though, I'm sure.
4. I'm feeling tremendously aroused sexually – but I have no idea why.
5. Oh! . . . (Silence.)

'Go on – tell me what you're thinking.'

6. I feel ashamed. Dreadfully ashamed. I remember now . . . I used to fantasize things like that to make it more exciting when I was playing with myself.
7. That explains a lot to me . . . (etc., etc.)

Again mark it 'Repression released – case closed'. Shall I go on? or am I boring you!

Sheer necessity dictates that from here on in, I am going to have to be a little disjointed with the writings. I have already sidetracked a lot, but it was only expediency, as I made the circular route into a jigsaw-puzzle picture for you. There is a picture there now for you to see – but in patches it is fuzzy and incomplete, and it is those grey areas that I will be darting among.

COUNTER-TRANSFERENCE

Unquestionably the greyest area remains in the realms of transference, which I have mentioned so often, and which is the kingpin around which the analysis pivots.

Again let me struggle to find words which do justice to the most profound of feelings. Firstly consider how fatuous is the remark: 'I know how you feel.' Nobody has any conception of how, and what, another person feels – in fact one of the megalomaniac symptoms of humans is to have the temerity to think that everybody thinks as they do, that everybody feels as they feel.

After a few sessions of analysis the analyst has, subconsciously, become somebody else to the client, somebody from that person's past. Usually he will not be aware of that consciously, although sometimes there will be instances where it consciously surfaces. A client brought me in a box of golf balls at session four/five as a token of affection/empathy. I just happened to say casually, 'What made you think I played golf, by the way?', which threw her into an 'almighty tizz'. She was visibly distressed and upset. She just did not know what had made her think I was a golfer. 'There is an "it" which thinks in me, and makes me doubt whether it is I that think . . .'. Of course, the subconscious had provided the information (I have not played for more than a decade, by the way) and that was why her intellect was so disturbed and upset – for a split second she almost had to ascribe her deepest emotions, wishes and desires to that intangible, unknowable, mental sphinx within herself.

No matter how hard you consciously try not to, your client's recollections will stir conscious and subconscious recollections in you of your own murky – sorry – blameless past.

After a few sessions of analysis the client has subconsciously – and I stress subconsciously – become somebody else to the analyst, somebody from that person's past. Usually the analyst will not be aware of that consciously, although sometimes there will be instances where it consciously surfaces. Have you read that before somewhere? Try back a couple of paragraphs or so – you need not hold it to the mirror to read it, though if I thought the printers could have coped, I would have written it that way. 'Counter transference' tends to mirror transference or, reworded, the analyst's way of dealing with the client tends to be a mirror of the way in which the client is dealing with the analyst.

Actually, you know, you can find out an awful lot of the problems the hard way – by practical experience – without either you or your clients coming to any harm. I confess I certainly did. I thought I understood transference from my own limited experience in analysis, but a few years later, with that miracle of illumination behind me – hindsight – I find that I did not really understand transference at all, and that I am only gradually coming to anything like a near total understanding of it now. The principal failing I want to save you and your clients from, is an unnecessary continuation of analysis – a person remaining in treatment on a search for subconscious anxiety, when it has ceased to be either necessary or, indeed, desirable that such a search should continue. When transference is complete, when it is total, so is the analysis. Dissolution of transference will then bring about the required internal change.

Dissolution of transference is the dissolving of a neurosis, because transference is, itself, neurotic. When an ice-cube dissolves and melts away, when the resultant water has dried and evaporated, there is nothing left to be seen of that artificially created ice-cube. It had appeared to be very strong and solid. It could create effects of its own, but dissolved it is a nothing, it is non-existent, it is not even there. In the case of transference, the neurosis from which it was spawned is also dissolved. The client who sends you a Christmas card expressing eternal gratitude is not totally cured. The client who discusses with you how wonderful analysis is, what a change it has wrought in him, how clear his insight, how total the cure, is not totally cured. Far from being his panacea, you have become his parasite – he has become slightly depersonalized by his seemingly harmless relationship with you – it is the last vestige of his neurosis adhering tenaciously. At the last moment of total dissolution, he will feel a final sensation of loss, as though some intangible, upon which he could depend and rely for support, had gone – leaving him lost – and then suddenly found. He finds himself, the person he was meant to be, prior to the intervention of fate. Try and explain this to him and you will invoke a similar reaction to that from an antitheist who, in his fervent opposition to the existence of God, cannot see that his very opposition is really a confirmation in itself – 'Tell me some more of this God in whom you do not believe.'

So how to decide when transference is complete? Well, there's the rub. The client cannot tell you. In a high percentage of cases it will not be necessary to decide, because the analysis will come to a focal point of release – a hefty repression released and understood, resulting in a natural conclusion to analysis, and an equally natural dissolution of transference. As the person hurriedly sets about disavowing what he has recalled, what he experienced to recall it, what had been wrong with him previously, and the one who had wrought all this – 'I don't think I was ever really that bad at all.'

Let us assume no tremendous focal point, perhaps plenty of emotion, session by session, plenty of recall, session by session, and the odd abstract thought to confuse the issue. There are as many possibilities now as legs on a centipede. Repressions do not have to be released in your consulting room. They are just as likely, no, somewhat more likely, to be released in the privacy of the person's own home. As he is dropping off to sleep, his mind wanders, 'imaginary' pictures flash into his mind, emotions get stirred – and a repression gets released. At the time of writing, a client 'told' me something, only as a routine sequence of recall, about a recollection from the past. He was somewhat ashamed in the telling of it, but it very obviously was not a repression, merely a bit of a disavowal – something he would have preferred not to think, or talk, about. Later in the session he was to confide that the recollection had been a repression and had assaulted his sensibilities, the night after he had been for his previous session.

He had even written in his diary under this day's date: 'Tell Mr F. the good news.' And yet it might easily have slipped by as of only minor consequence. The consequences of it slipping by unnoticed? Still in the grip of transference the client would retain his indirect symptoms. We could have gone on looking for the point of release for weeks; it would have needed me to observe that transference was complete, was total, and, in consequence, to discharge the person from treatment. Whereupon he would have no alternative but to dissolve the transference – however long it takes. Bear in mind that you, the therapist, the analyst, cannot dissolve transference for your client – he can only do that for himself.

Now that sounds easy enough, doesn't it? Just simply ascertain when transference is total and discharge the person from treatment. It would work perfectly with androids! We, of course, have that notorious intangible to reckon with – the human element. Problem one: to decide when transference really is total. Problem two: to discharge an apparently uncured person from treatment – 'I'm sure I'll remember soon . . . I've got faith in you . . . I can afford it . . . I'll come next week.'

How do you overcome these intangibles? Well, again I feel like fatuously remarking 'with the greatest of difficulty'. Seriously, though, you will find a way. Personally, I make sure that control is always in my court. I declare in my paperwork that analysis takes between five and eight sessions at weekly intervals; that if analysis is necessary beyond session eight, then it continues at either half normal fee or without fee at all; and that, at session thirteen, the person would be automatically discharged from treatment. I know, from practical experience, that a small percentage of my clients will be like homing pigeons, and that my attitudes have to be totally flexible, and with no hard and fast rules at all. However, I reiterate that it is good policy to have an apparently resolute pattern, itemized in publicity material, or on waiting-room walls. As I have said before, strictly speaking there is no such thing as a failed analysis – only in degree. One session of analysis is ultimately of benefit to the person, however slight. I might have hinted at it jokingly, but I really mean what I say: Many times a person will discharge himself from treatment, or you will discharge him from treatment –

only to find that with the dissolution of transference comes a complete or partial cure. The person's attitude? 'I realized when he couldn't do anything for me that I just had to help myself and sort out my own life – I feel fantastic now – only wish I hadn't wasted all that money.'

I have a letter I prize above all others: 'I consulted you with an inferiority complex and fear of sex, but have decided not to waste any more money with you. I've been thinking about this inferior thing, and I don't honestly think it is me; it's probably everybody else, and as far as sex is concerned, I think it is probably the nicest thing in the world.' Remember also that I said it took a special, or rather, unusual, sort of personality to be an analyst. I very seldom take my work home, but that particular letter I told my wife about, and she was most indignant: 'Write to him. Tell him, make him realize that you have cured him.' She was quite annoyed that I was so complacently amused by it. I did say I was quite prepared to content myself with being right, though, didn't I – and so I am.

SYMPTOM FORMATION AND ALTERATION

Analysis sets out to bring a person to a point of enlightenment which frees him from his hang-ups and brings about an internal change within himself.

The actual symptoms put forward by the person are not really – or not only – the problem that analysis sets out to resolve; they are only what are called 'presenting symptoms' which have been brought about by a conflict within the psyche of that person. Analysis sets out to recreate that original conflict all over again, to revive it, and to dissolve it. The person's maturity, experience, and changed sense of values will deal effortlessly with a juvenile conflict – once the conflict is realized, appreciated and understood by the person.

People's presenting symptoms change through the years. A perfect example of this is in the realms of phobias, where the presenting phobia is frequently only a substitution (often many times removed – almost to the power of *n*) of the original phobia, and the original phobia is only a substitution, a symbolic representation, of the original conflict. I think I can illustrate this for you so that you can understand more clearly what I am trying to say.

Let us take, as an example, a little girl who wets herself in front of all her classmates, and is at the receiving end of a lot of taunts and teasing. She is going to start taking precautions to make sure such a thing never happens again. She will go for a wee before she leaves for school, she will go for a wee at the beginning of break, towards the end of break, before dinner, after dinner, twice in the afternoon break – and, just to be on the safe side, one more wee before she sets off for home. Coué's law of reversed effort is, of course, going to make sure that yet another puddle appears under her desk before too long – to her intense mortification. There is every chance now that the incidents will succumb to repression. That being the case, she will be left with a 'compulsive activity' – the interminable visits to the loo – without intellectually knowing why. She will likely attest to a weak bladder for the rest of her life. The visits to the loo will serve to ward off 'the unknown'. She will have a fear of wetting herself in public – but will not know *why* she has such a fear, the originating incidents and emotions being concealed from her by the repression process. That is part one of my illustration: the development of the original phobia and the birth of the original anxiety. Realize that she is going to be a bit of a psychological mess in later life, although no more so than the rest of a sick humanity 'whose suffering afflicts us all' (Jung). She will have subconscious guilt about urinating, menstruating (producing premenstrual tension), indeed about sex itself, and I will bet she has the greatest difficulty in climaxing, no matter what stimulus she receives.

Now, into part two of my illustration: a phobia has to be appropriate, it has to serve a purpose – to guard against, to ward off, the unknown; that nameless, formless, timeless, free-floating abstract within the person. At the same time it has to satisfy intellect, which is the thing that intrudes to create the symbolic interpretation. As our girl example matures, the actual chances of her wetting herself in public recede, and recede so as to become most unlikely. The phobia is getting 'worked out' – so it will change. Symbolism will dictate the new one, but it will probably have a vague connection – say a fear of vomiting (which is also an emission from a bodily orifice) in public. That is going to have a manifold purpose too, of hitting her where it hurts her most – which is that sneaky habit the mind has got – by making it a nightmare for her to accept a dinner date. That, of course, effectively stops her having to 'sing for her supper', as the saying goes, which in turn satisfies the inhibition in the sexuality.

The processes involved are immensely complex and intertwined, and my over-simplification is there to be shot at; nevertheless, at base roots, that is roughly what happens.

In analysis she will recreate the original conflict – it will be touch and go whether she wets my couch or not at the moment of recall. What would perhaps happen in practice, in a case like that, the person would usually remember the originating incidents rather vaguely, experience a degree of shame during the session . . . and then have to break off the session to go to the toilet. That night, though, I would not like to sleep in the same bed with her. The originating memory is almost certain to force itself upon her emotions, and also likely to force itself upon her physically, in the form of an abreaction. That will teach her moaning husband a lesson, for begrudging the cost of my fees, though, won't it?

All we set out to do was to revive the actual memory; to re-create the original conflict. But – as we get closer and closer to the conflict – the person tends to get more and more anxious. Now, of course, her anxiety is focalized: upon the analysis – so her general anxieties in life, her phobias, stutters, twitches, rashes, etc., do tend to have their sting taken out of them, their intensity subdued.

Let us recall again the stutterer from Chapter 7. In the week leading up to his final session, he would likely have got a vague thought present itself to his consciousness, the nagging doubts he had about his own sexuality would have become almost concrete fears. He would 'feel' that the likely outcome of analysis was to 'prove' that he really was gay and that he would have to resign himself to that 'fact'. The closer and closer he came to releasing the repressed recollection – the more and more convinced he would become that his worst fears were to be realized. Until . . . the moment of release . . . he sees his childhood dread for what it really is: a childhood dread. In that moment of insight the fear evaporates, and his heterosexuality is assured. I wish I had a pound for every time a client has said something akin to the following to me about half-way through analysis: 'I feel almost as though I've committed a terrible crime but I have no idea what it is.'

Herein lies the fallacy of the old motto, 'Let sleeping dogs lie.' The dogs we set out to disturb were already restless, growling, and grumbling, long before we came upon the scene. Our prying and prodding stirs them up, so they start to bark and bite at the person who is stirring them up; but then we open the cage and let them out – and they wouldn't go back in the cage even if they could.

The memories brought to light in analysis, the recall of the repressed material or emotions – they are not all of it; in fact, they are not the half of it. The cure, the internal change is only part-way achieved by recall; the major part is transference. That is the agent which ensures the change – the creation of and the dissolution of, an emotional tie to the analyst. No transference – no cure . . . transference remains – problem remains . . . transference gone – problem gone. The transference re-creates old feelings, emotions, and psychological experiences and desires and attaches them to the analyst. A certain group of people cannot do this, though, while another group of people are likely to do it far too strongly.

NARCISSISM

The group who cannot fulfil 'transference' remain forever beyond the reach of analysis – they will have to find their help from the hands, or rather advices, of the behaviour therapists, or more traditional psychiatry. In analysis they will remain indifferent to the analyst; not by conscious decision, but by unconscious choice. So who are these inward-turning people? It's all right, you can relax; it was a rhetorical question. These inward-turning people are the ones whose neuroses are totally inward – what is termed 'narcissistic'. Remember Narcissus? He and I went to different schools together, and he was the one who looked in the lake and fell in love with his own reflection, although the odd bit of pomposity in these writings makes me suspect I caught a tiny peek, too. However . . . narcissistic neuroses are so inward turned . . . the original happening, person or emotion, so lost to him, so concealed by repression, time and substitution that the person is incapable of transference, and therefore not amenable to analysis. How do you recognize such people? (Rhetorical questions are coming thick and fast now.) Well, again I could be fatuous: 'With the greatest of . . .' – but that would dodge the question. The easiest way, of course, to recognize such people, is with –

hindsight, that illuminator extraordinary. It is easy to observe when a person is in the grip of transference, and equally easy to observe when he is not. In any case, not having fallen into the grip of transference, the narcissistic sufferer will find no merit at all in analysis and will withdraw by session three or, at the latest, session four. To recognize this group at first meeting is somewhat more difficult. They usually have a habit of picking others up on what they say – in circumstances where normal politeness would allow the comment to go unchallenged. They are usually self-opinionated, self-centred and selfish, and at the same time very sorry for themselves, often remorseless in their self-criticism, but always using it as self-justification.

HOMOSEXUALITY

Homosexuality usually, but by no means always, is a narcissistic neurosis. The person he really wants to make love to is himself – he just cannot get round to it. I would never offer to transform a person's homosexuality to heterosexuality – not that they would want me to, anyway, but I would always warn the homosexual who was attending for analysis, say for a stutter, that the likely outcome of a successful analysis would be to reverse his homosexuality. Homosexuals, of both sexes, are the only group of people to whom I make any such explanation prior to analysis (presupposing they have disclosed their homosexuality to me). The only reason I predict such an outcome when they consult me with nerve rashes, migraines, stutters, premature ejaculation, phobias, or what you will, is because I am firstly a realist. The business of living is not all beer and candy-floss, and joint mortgages, business partnerships, shared leases, and the great god money, all have their devastating influences upon us all. I consider it morally necessary for me to forewarn the homosexual. The fact that either: (a) he totally disbelieves me, (b) he takes fright and decides to go elsewhere for treatment, or (c) he remains open-minded as to the outcome – none of these reactions bother me. Should he proceed in analysis I write on the front of his notes: 'I have been told one of the likely results of analysis will be to restore my heterosexuality' – and I get him to sign it. (I don't want to get involved in any possible lawsuit between him and his 'affair', so I protect myself.) Naturally I am aware that a high percentage of homosexuals will be incapable of transference and consequently immune to analysis. But I don't know with the particular individual sat in front of me whether or not that applies.

Broadly speaking, homosexuality is of far more concern to the individual when it is 'latent' rather than 'blatant'. The homosexual is well content with that state – rather like the sadist and the masochist, they enjoy their deviation. I will never forget a professional man, standing in my doorway subsequent to his last session of analysis, saying to me, 'I just cannot find it in my heart to thank you. I honestly feel that you have taken something from me.' He had consulted me, solely for his wife's sake, to be cured of his sado-masochistic tendencies which involved canes and wire hairbrushes at bedtime – but, in the cure, he realized that his 'pleasures once perceived' were gone.

When, however, these deviations are latent and concealed from a person's intellectual awareness, then the effect upon their psyche is far more damaging. Again, remember that they will be vehement in their denials: 'I couldn't stand another woman to touch me, even shaking hands with a woman I find difficult,' says the latent lesbian. Repressions have got that peculiar trick of inversion – like being passed through the lens of a camera – the effect gets turned inside out and/or upside down. Anal eroticism is a classic example, spawned in the young years; the pleasures of passing faeces can remain as a desire for pleasure from touch of the anal passage, or it can be vigorously rejected by the juvenile mind, and the ability to experience pleasure via sensation with the anal passage becomes repressed. A repression produces a symptom, remember! Likely symptom (1): 'I couldn't stand anybody to touch my anal passage, I think it's revolting, just the thought of it makes me feel sick.' Likely symptom (2): 'I like to pinch or bite when I'm having sex, I can't help it, it is just something I do.' (Anal eroticism, latent or blatant, originates from the anal/sadistic period of development, remember, so is easily distorted into sadism.)

Using a similar analogy to that of the camera lens, these repressions – producing inversions – can produce projections: the guy who likes to put his finger into his partner's anal passage whilst having sex, subconsciously wants his partner to do the same to his anal passage. Discuss it with him (not at the dinner table, please) and he would vehemently deny your insinuation and would profess, 'Oh no! I'd hate it – I like doing it though – I can't think why – I just like it.' The subconscious projection/inversion could be far more insidious than the example I have given though, and could indicate the presence of latent homosexuality.

ABBREVIATED ANALYSIS

Generally speaking, I am not advocating total analysis for your client. That rather sweeping statement needs some amplification or it will sound as though I am advocating inadequate treatment for the person.

View analysis as a progressive thing. Assume we are trying to get from point A to point Z. We may well settle for point K, or point R, or some other midway point that has achieved a purpose. Understand this: if we reach point Z then the person has remembered being born – the trauma of birth itself – not imagined it, but remembered it. Understand, too, that the presence of a repression within a person puts obstacles in the way of all their recall around that period of development when the repression occurred; that does not mean they cannot remember other incidents around this time, it means it is more difficult for them to remember other incidents around this time. Common sense tells you that if you can remove the repression you also clear the way to the other recall. Logically following that line of discussion shows you that removing one repression will clear the way towards releasing an earlier repression, and so on.

OK, that's clear enough, surely. However, let us once again drag back our defiled ex-stutterer, who serves as such a good illustrator. Remember I said that when he had released the repression to do with the man in the brown suit, I did some checking to make sure there was not an associated repression. Well, bear with me for a moment and I will explain, and if, in the explanation, I sound rather ruthless – well, I did use the word 'unusual' about the analyst's character.

When the client released that repressed recollection, he was very emotional, he was very upset, hovering on the verge of being physically sick, and a humanitarian attitude would appear to demand words of comfort and reassurance from his therapist. What did he get instead? He got me checking for associated repressions. Doesn't sound too bad, does it? I bet you would not like to have been at the receiving end of it, feeling as he felt then. Instead of that 'comfort and reassurance' he got a verbal slanging, said with a lot of venom and with a high degree of emotion. I accused him in no uncertain manner of having sat at the tea table, looking at his dad, and wondering what it would be like if his dad did the same. I forcibly drew his attention to the fact that one of his earlier recollections of analysis had been of his dad holding him up in the water by his swimming trunks when teaching him to swim – perhaps he had wanted his dad to pull them down like the man did. His emotions were already reeling under the effects of the release of the repression . . . now they were in tatters. Whether any of my verbal arrows (huh! cannonballs!) got through to him, I honestly don't know – and care even less. He paid me to do a job of work and I did it to the best of my ability.

Minus the repression to do with the brown suit, it would have been fairly easy to continue for another four or five sessions when, almost certainly, the Oedipus complex would have been released from repression, and then to start again for a few more sessions until potty-training repressions were released, and then to continue for some more sessions until 'oral' conflicts and their repressions were released, and finally to continue for some more sessions until birth trauma was released. One thing that the release of a repression, particularly from yourself, does convince you, is that there must be others lurking.

Now I have taken people the whole route (which would, by inference, tend to disprove Jung's statement that one cannot take anybody to a stage further than you have reached yourself), but the number of times I have helped anyone to those lengths is somewhat limited.

In my own opinion the Oedipal, anal, oral and birth repressions are the ones that are common to mankind, and by the way of symptoms, create nothing worse than the 'suffering which afflicts us all'. Should one of them be creating 'abnormal' symptoms, due to a more hefty bite at the cherry, then by all means let us dig for it. Should the client have access to sufficient time, money, effort and self-discipline (as well as having sufficient enthusiasm) to delve that deep – again, by all means let's do it. Otherwise we will settle for a bit of evolution rather than total revolution.

Perhaps I ought to add a proviso to the foregoing. Earlier I said that symptoms had to be judged in relationship to environmental pressures, and that the most neurotic person would remain comparatively stable if the environment remained kind, whereas the most rational person would break down if the pressures were enough. So, my proviso is this: the greater the pressure a person is to be subjected to, the greater the need for extended analysis. At the risk of a lawsuit I will give you a couple of examples, probably two of the most famous people of recent decades – Marilyn Monroe and Elvis Presley – both of whom brought themselves to a tragic and untimely end. Look at those two stars through the eyes of a psychoanalyst, and their lifestyles demonstrate quite clearly that they had both taken an above-average bite from the Oedipal cherry. Had the pressures of the environment been more normal for the luckless pair – had Monroe remained in a waitress's uniform, her attraction to the more mature male would have had only minor psychological effects upon her; had Presley remained behind the wheel of a truck, then he would likely only have bored his spouse by insisting on going to his mother's every Sunday. In both their cases the tremendous pressures of the environment they chose, or rather which chose them, caused those subconscious forces to exert an ever more and more savage effect upon them.

Before you dismiss the foregoing as far-fetched, think about it. I am going to content myself with thinking that, on the preponderance of probabilities, I am right. In both cases, of course, they had access to the best medical brains that money can buy . . . need I say more. 'Where matters of the mind are concerned, you may be assured that all doctors are laymen, and that certainly includes most psychiatrists.'

9.
AN INTRODUCTION TO HYPNOSIS

I am now going to explain something about the hypnotic phenomenon. Elsewhere we have agreed that an idea which takes root in the subconscious must be discharged in motor action to the individual – but since the motivation then comes from the subconscious, it naturally follows that the person is not intellectually aware of the subconscious motivation taking place. That sounds awfully complicated; perhaps it is just the way I have expressed it. I will try again. A person acting as a result of a subconscious idea does not know why he is doing what he is doing. There, that has expressed it more simply. But what does that mean from a practical viewpoint? Well, when you give someone a post-hypnotic suggestion, which does take root in the subconscious, the person is going to act upon that suggestion — but of course he will not know why he is doing whatever it is he is doing (or not doing, as the case may be). He will most likely attempt to rationalize his actions and will never willingly attribute them to your post-hypnotic suggestion – even if he ever connects the two, which again is more unlikely. Although the person will usually remember the post-hypnotic suggestion having been given to him, he will still not realize he is acting upon it.

Bring what I have said down to a silly example. Give someone a post-hypnotic suggestion to the effect that when dressing he is to put his shoes on the wrong feet. Should the suggestion take root in the subconscious, it must be discharged – the person will put his shoes dutifully on the wrong feet. Ask him why, and he will have a most involved and complicated explanation, probably to the effect that the shoes were tight on the sides, and it seemed a good way of stretching them – he will not willingly admit to himself, let alone you, that he is acting under post-hypnotic suggestion, because he will not know he is. Again, he will probably remember the suggestion but disavow that it has had any affect upon his actions.

Should you ever get the chance to talk to a volunteer from a stage hypnosis show, do so. Listen to him explain why he carried out the silly tasks – and marvel at man's self-deception. Go a step further and you will find that most people do not want to think that they even entered the hypnotic state at all, let alone altered their actions as a result.

From a practical point of view, this means you're skating on thin ice if you want to ram it down your client's throat: (a) that he has been hypnotized, or (b) that his actions, thoughts or motivations are a result of your post-hypnotic sugges n. To be frank, it should not matter to you anyway. Yet again you can content yourself with being right, and there is just no need to prove the client wrong. You are meant to be helping him in life, not triumphing over him. Should you be the sort of person who needs thanks, recognition and acknowledgement of what you are doing, then you have embarked on the wrong course here; because, as a very general statement of fact, your clients are going to say that they were never really that bad, that they never needed to go to you in the first place. Remember the letter I prize which reads: 'I consulted you with an inferiority complex and fear of sex, but have decided not to waste any more money with you. I've been thinking about this inferior thing, and I don't honestly think it is me; it's probably everybody else – and as far as sex is concerned, I think it's probably the nicest thing in the world.'

I can think of no reason at all for a therapist needing to prove the hypnotic state to his client. It must only be to satisfy his own ego. The idea of a trained therapist indulging in what are no more than cheap vaudeville tricks with a client, merely to prove to the person that he is in hypnosis, leaves me wanting only to take the therapist into analysis to find out why. I recently watched a doctor on TV pass a needle through the flesh of a hypnotized subject to prove she felt no pain. He could never convince me that his motives were other than egotistical. Do your explaining about the hypnotic state before you ever commence therapy, and thereafter simply be reassuring with respect to the client's doubts and worries.

We all pass through the hypnotic state at least twice a day; once upon waking, and again upon retiring. That lethargic state one feels on a Sunday morning when, with your eyes still closed, you think to yourself, 'Shall I wake up or not?' – knowing full well that you are already awake. That feeling is as deserving of the title 'hypnogogic', as is the state produced by a stage performer upon a volunteer participator. I will state here and now, quite categorically, something I believe to be true – a belief which no one could destroy: the only person above the age of about eight years, who cannot be hypnotized, is a mental defective (with the only other exception being the heavily inebriated person or drug 'tripper' – and in both these cases I would not, of course, attempt an induction). Having carried out tens of thousands of inductions, across every age group and strata of society, I find it impossible to concede the slightest doubt at all, but that the induction will be successful. The degree of acceptance of hypnosis will vary from person to person. When I hear people say, 'I went to a hypnotist but he couldn't get me under,' I marvel only at the lack of knowledge of the science the hypnotist is using, or rather sometimes misusing. There is no such thing as a 'hypnotized feeling', so the subject is in no position to judge whether he is hypnotized or not. The hypnotist, or independent observer, can clearly evaluate the existence of the hypnotic phenomenon, so long as he knows what to look for and knows what he is doing. I say again, that if a hypnotic induction is carried out on a consenting person (and sometimes even on an apparently non-consenting person – but I'll touch on that later), then provided that person is not mentally defective, provided he is not at the time heavily under the effects of alcohol or drugs, then that person will enter the hypnotic state. Please let me stress that I am not saying that he will necessarily know that he is in the hypnotic state, nor yet will he necessarily know afterwards that he had been in the hypnotic state; once again, I shall merely content myself with knowing that I am right.

Let me illustrate the point I am trying to get across.

WAKING HYPNOSIS

A dentist decides to remove a tooth from his client and tells him so. He then dips a piece of cotton-wool into a small flask of cold water and says to the person, 'This is a particularly strong anaesthetic. It freezes in less than fifteen seconds. Will you please signal when it has frozen your gum.' He then dabs the bad tooth and the gum around the bad tooth with the cold-water-impregnated swab, and waits expectantly . . . . Within the allotted fifteen seconds the client would affirm that the gum had frozen. The dental nurse could then be asked to inspect and attest the fact that the gum area was white and frozen. It would be! As well and truly frozen as ever cocaine could have done.

Here we are, or rather the dentist is, using a phenomenon known as 'waking hypnosis'. A psychosomatic effect has been produced by pure suggestion. Should the dentist then proceed to tell the client that he had been hoaxed, and prove this by drinking from the cold water, the gum would immediately unfreeze.

A lot of what we have been learning about was at work in that dentist's surgery. The client was, without doubt, paying attention to what was going on, so a prerequisite of hypnosis was already present. The subject was given a suggestion to act upon; an idea was to take root in the subconscious – and consequently must be discharged in motor action. Emile Coué popped in to make sure the imagination was at work; the conscious will was defeated – mind reacted upon body, body reacted upon mind. Job done. There were little extras to help it along: well, he certainly looked like a dentist and the client certainly was in a dentist's chair. What the dentist said did not exactly leave room for doubt. The 'anaesthetic' surely was cold. The patient was in an emotionally charged state, and could see no reason to doubt.

That client now happily and painlessly minus a tooth, was hypnotized – yes he was! (Go back and look at my original definition.) Is the dentist going to tell him so? And if he does do you think his technique will be very successful next time with that same client? A percentage of dentists actually do work in the way I have described; other dentists would say, 'Oh, I have studied hypnosis but it is too protracted and time-consuming.' I would merely think, 'Then you have not studied hypnosis either enough or at all.'

I hope my little anecdote about your friendly neighbourhood dentist has turned upside-down, or at least altered, any preconceptions (and probably misconceptions) you may have had on the subject of hypnosis.

LAW OF AVERAGES

Now I want to try and turn those same misconceptions inside out. A stage performer calls for volunteers to be hypnotized, and gets, say, twenty or thirty mixed sexes and age groups onto the stage. Here, by the way, I speak with some insight, as I have – to my eternal shame, and many years ago now – done some stage performing with hypnosis. He carries out a couple of quick tests of 'suggestibility' on the volunteers, and mentally selects the ones most likely to participate wholeheartedly in the fun. Then he carries out a quick induction technique aimed at all the volunteers, but paying particular attention to the ones he has mentally singled out. Every single one of the volunteers will enter the hypnotic state – to a greater or lesser degree, but, of course, they will not know that. (Indeed, unless his studies have been thorough, even the hypnotist himself will not have realized that he has been so successful.) Within minutes he will be sending back to their seats the least suggestible of the subjects, they proudly announcing to all and sundry that their mind 'must have been too strong for him' or other such pathetic human assertion. One by one he will return subjects to the audience until he is left with a controllable number, say about seven to ten (dependent upon his skills of memory, manipulation and sheer force of character). These, more suggestible, more co-operative, fun seekers, he will use to give his performance proper.

I met a salesman once who believed so implicitly in statistics and the law of averages that he was totally convinced that each working day of his life he would meet two 'bastards' and one 'nice guy'. He used this formula to make an extremely good income, selling, on average, to one in three of the persons he told his story to – that is the one he called the 'nice guy'.

A law of averages also seems to exist within hypnosis, inasmuch as a group of thirty subjects will usually yield, on average, one somnambulist. Now a somnambulist for our purposes is not a sleepwalker, but rather a person who will go to the deeper states of hypnosis when the state is suggested to him. His recall of events taking place during the session will afterwards be rather vague, and during the session he will demonstrate the appearance of a trance-like state. In therapy his deep acceptance of the hypnotic phenomenon is nothing short of a nuisance – and to a stage performer he can also be a bit of a pain, preferring to 'sleep' his way through a session, rather than participating in the various demonstrations.

The ability of a person to accept suggestion is, of course, decided in his forming years. It is yet another of his predispositions. It is difficult to give examples of causes of predisposition to suggestibility, but if you take the example of the parent who is always telling a child: 'Now if you do – such and such a thing, then – such and such will happen'; 'If you wash you hands and face now, Father Christmas will bring you a bike' – these sorts of suggestions to a child would most likely render him less and less predisposed to accepting suggestions, particularly if those parental threats and promises had usually proved abortive.

During his performance, the stage performer is going to persuade his volunteers to carry out various amusing acts for the benefit of the audience. The audience will presume that the subjects are in some sort of trance; that they have no awareness of what they are doing or why they are doing it; that they have no alternative but to carry out the appointed tasks, and that afterwards they will not be aware of what has taken place. Boloney! There is no such thing as a 'hypnotized feeling', so none of the subjects thought they were hypnotized. Each, with the exception perhaps of the somnambulist, was well aware of what was taking place. They thought that their own reasons for carrying out the appointed tasks when asked to were perfectly reasonable reasons (usually to the effect that, having volunteered to make a fool of themselves on stage, it would have been embarrassing to decline to do the things, and so make a fool of the hypnotist); and that their recall of the entire show was total. There are, of course, more forces at work than they realize, but for all that, their thoughts are not so inaccurate.

Please, please, please do not run away with the idea that I am belittling hypnosis – 'it' is a most amazing phenomenon, and offers considerable potential for the improvement of the human lot. I am making the point that it is not as most people believe it to be. It is certainly non-magical, and is a naturally occurring phenomenon. Subject to you having understood and absorbed that which I have so far explained, then you should be able to understand most of the forces at work in hypnosis. There will always remain an intangible. I am reminded of that satirical joke which says that just one word will destroy the most sophisticated computer known to man's ingenuity: simply program the computer with the question 'Why?' In these writings I am endeavouring to explain much about man's behaviour – the conscious and unconscious causes at work – in the hope that you will view your own, and your clients', thought patterns in a different light. I shall mostly stay well clear of metaphysical matters. Even so, I would like to make just one point: Jung, who was originally a disciple of Freud and who broke away from Freud to formulate his own differing theories, made much of the 'collective unconscious' – meaning, in a way, the idea that there is not just you, and there is not just me, there is also subconsciously *us*. This puts across the idea of us all having access to the same subconscious knowledge – rather like thinking of the ant hill as a living entity with its own digestive tract, its own excretion process, its own repairing process, and so on, and, thinking of the ants merely as cells of life within the hill, rather than thinking of them being only individuals in their own right. Even if I had the words to express my own beliefs on such subjects I would not want to do so here; instead I would like you to carry out the following experiment with friends, acquaintances and relatives.

SYMBOLISM

Take a piece of paper and divide it in two with a line drawn from top to bottom. Write the letter H on the top of the left-hand side, and the letter L on the top of the right-hand side. Tell your subject that you want him to express something in symbolic form on the paper with the pencil you are providing. You want him, without using words, to illustrate the word you use. Now get your subject poised with pencil in hand, waiting to put something into the left-hand column – say that you want him to do it quickly, and without giving it a lot of thought. Next say to the subject that you are ready, that you want him to symbolize this word on the paper, as soon as you say it, and the word you want him to symbolize is – Hate! That is it – Hate! Go on, put some Hate! on the paper. As soon as he has marked the paper in some way, thank him and then say that you also want him to symbolize something in the other column of the paper. Again, get him poised with the pencil and the paper; now say that you want him to express – Love! Yes, Love! Love! Onto the paper, you want him to symbolize Love! on the paper. As soon as he has marked the paper, again thank him, and now produce your previously completed master copy, made up as in Figure 4.

Figure 4 — Master copy

You are going to find, in all probability, that his symbols are very similar to your masters – although, at first glance they may appear different. Hate, for example, may have been drawn as in Figure 5, but are they really so very different? All demonstrate abrupt angles and changes of direction.

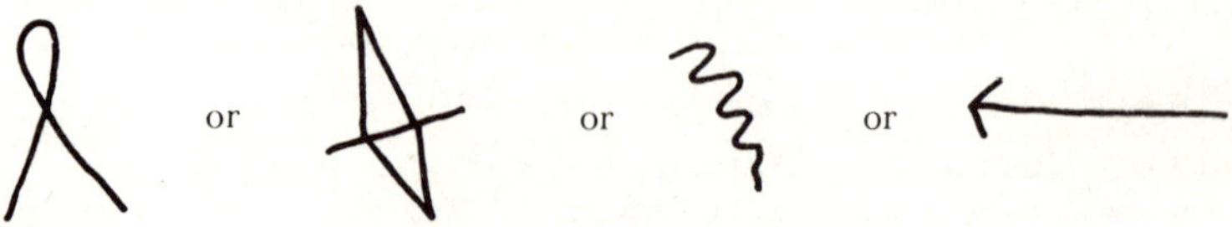

Figure 5 — Hate symbols

Love may have been symbolized as shown in Figure 6, but again, are they different at all? Or is the same basic shape present?

Figure 6 — Love symbols

Try it. Try it again and yet again. Try it on a Latvian, a Peruvian, an African, a German, or any nationality on this planet. When you have proved, to your entire satisfaction, that we do tend to symbolize in the same way – then risk blowing up your computer by asking why?

The waters into which I have barely dipped a toe run very deep, and I have no intention of getting wet. I am going a very long-winded way round to say that if you want perfection in what you do, if you need to know all the answers, and all the reasons, then switch to mathematical formulae and cease concerning yourself with the human psyche. Your client will enter your door as a very fallible human being, and, pursuant to your treatment, he will depart your door still very much a fallible human being. You may well have helped him considerably in his life, but he still is, and will forever remain, a fallible human being. Nobody, but nobody, ever becomes utterly qualified, utterly intelligent and utterly successful in achieving everything he sets out to do.

Staying with the subject of hypnosis, I now want to move away from dentistry or stage performance, and think of the application to our therapy. The scientific approach to hypnosis has discovered some quite remarkable things about many people in the hypnotic state, such as the drop in electrical resistance across the surface of the skin (bio-feedback meters have much to tell us here, as well) and the increase in audio reception to their normally more dormant hearing side. Many scientists speak of the different spheres of the brain and discuss how hypnosis allows a freer flow of information between them. What I, in turn, could show them about hypnosis is hampered by a blindfolding gag, because it just cannot be demonstrated.

Using the hypnotic state as an aid to encourage rapport between therapist and client, as an aid to permit exchange of confidence, and finally as an aid to bring about a release from the client's inner anxiety, demands privacy. It demands the establishment of a relationship between client and therapist whereby the client knows that his confidences will not be breached. The material sought by analysis will not come anywhere near his conscious thoughts until such time as a very special relationship has been struck between the two; not until such time as the phenomenon of transference is complete. The moment it is suggested a third party should observe, or that a client should be connected to monitoring equipment, or that the session should be taped or filmed or otherwise recorded – that moment would bring analysis crashing to an abrupt and sudden full stop. The person will yield the information required; in fact the information required will only become available to him, as a result of having already confided the most intimate of his thoughts, wishes and desires, to another.

The phenomenon which occurs is provable, of course, but only to one person at a time – normally, each client. He will find it equally impossible, even if he should wish to do so, to convince a doubting humanity of the truth which he had experienced. I have already been obliged to comment wryly that, 'there is no court to appeal to'. Nobody, not you or I can possibly imagine how we would be, if we were not as we are. We can have no conception of the internal change which will be wrought by analysis – indeed, a lot of it we will not even notice, except with the advantage of hindsight. What chance, then, for example, of convincing a 'friend at the pub' that his dreadful fear of injections is likely to be latent homosexuality, or that his horror of dentists is potentially a repressed castration complex. No therapist in his right senses would allow the conversation even to veer in that direction, and would hastily interpose comments about the state of the world recession. (Herein lies the reason why the writings of Freud and others – indeed, in their turn, these writings – have intellectual criticism heaped upon them.) Our friend in the pub would react with indignation at our insinuations, in fact, he would likely overreact. Why? Because subconsciously he knows your allegations are true, and you would, unwittingly, have 'touched a subconscious nerve' and our protesting Cassius will not thank you for it.

Perhaps I appear to be labouring the difficulties a little; if I do, it is only because the difficulties really are enormous. Analysis clearly cannot be demonstrated, and just as clearly cannot be explained in a few hundred words. Probably a better way of tackling this problem would be the following: get your client to lie down in a warm room and close his eyes. Talk reassuringly to him for about ten minutes, and then ask him to say the very first thing that comes into his head and to keep saying whatever does come into his thoughts for about the next three-quarters of an hour. Do this at approximately weekly intervals for about six or seven weeks and the client will come to a realization and release of his problems.

If nothing else, it has saved a lot of paper and a lot of

writing. As a statement it is probably just about as believable – or unbelievable, as the case may be – to doubting, questioning ears.

PARAPSYCHOLOGY

Despite the overwhelming evidence to the contrary, many people believe that using hypnosis can make a person do something they do not want to do. Professional and amateur hypnotists come from all strata of society, and of course are not confined to one particular character type – within our three definitions of character type. The paranoidal mentality, with its desire to exploit others, is very likely to try his hand at being Svengali. Man is really rather a credulous animal (there goes my cynicism again) and stuffed to the gills with absurd, magical beliefs, which have not really changed all that much since the days when he copulated in the wheat fields to make sure the crops grew, or urinated on the meadow to ensure rain, or prayed to one of his gods for help and assistance. The paranoidal mentality is even more inclined towards such mysticism than the rest of humanity, and will often look for proof of the existence of magic, the black arts, or supernatural phenomena. Hypnosis to such people epitomizes the 'unknown', and they will forever be searching for new magical happenings and, because they have no understanding of the forces they are misusing, they will take at face value what they observe. A typical example would be the phenomenon known as 'pre-natal regression' – the idea of regressing a person, in the hypnotic state, back to a 'past life' experience which, in common with ouija boards, seances and the like, is really doing nothing more than tapping the subconscious layers of the mind of one or more of the participants. The dangers of deception and self-deception are enormous.

The idea of past life regression has received a lot of publicity, and from mankind's point of view it would be very satisfying to discover it to be true. After all, if you can find out you lived a previous life, you ought to be fairly confident of living a future one. The professional gambler would always bet on future life rather than against it, but of course his motives are suspect. He looks only at the odds – should he lose he does not have to pay out, and should he win, he collects.

Well, I hope you are sitting comfortably, because I'm sorry, folks – I do not believe that there is any such thing as 'pre-natal regression' within the hypnotic experience. I know many people would disagree with me, but I consider them to be wrong. The phenomenon is explainable; even when the subject has spoken in a language alien to his conscious knowledge (that is called xenoglossia, by the way) it is still explainable. But surely by now you are not that surprised – did I not say that every facet of human behaviour was explainable?

The world's authority on the subject of past life regression is one Dr Ian Stevenson, one-time Carlson Professor of Psychiatry, University of Virginia, USA, and he became a world authority on the subject by the obvious expedient of doing a lot – and I mean a lot – of research into it. Naturally, he is not the only one to have looked into it; Dr Roger A. Strauss of the University of California, and many other eminent men have extensively investigated it, but Dr Stevenson is universally acknowledged to have acquired the most experience of the phenomenon – probably due to the size of the financial grant his faculty awarded to the subject.

Dr Stevenson has published his views for all to read and he makes it very clear that he entirely disapproves of any such experiments – which I suppose is slightly unfair of him really as he, over several thousand cases, has 'had his fun', as it were. However, his motives for his present-day stance appear honest enough. He makes the point that the hypnotically evoked 'previous personality' may be extremely plausible – both to the person having the experience and to the hypnotist and others observing. The subject may produce surprisingly accurate historical detail, or lapse into a foreign tongue, which he cannot speak in his more normal day-to-day state of mind. The 'previous personality' may experience quite dramatic and emotional happenings, but Dr Stevenson concluded that although the subject quite frequently could not recall where he might possibly have obtained all this information within this life, it is nevertheless possible to utilize the hypnotic state to go searching for the subject's source of material, which, surprise, surprise, is his books, TV programmes, films, radio, etc. Dr Stevenson was also at some pains to point out that this type of regression is not without some danger, as instances have occurred where the evoked 'previous personality' has not 'gone away' when instructed to do so, and the subject has been left in an altered state for several days. Dr Stevenson concluded by saying that he was no longer conducting such experiments, that he was no longer interested in attempting to verify other hypnotists' apparent regressions, that he does not approve of any hypnotist making promises to clients that they will return to a previous life, and that he certainly does not approve of anyone charging fees for acting as a hypnotist in such experiments.

Neither Dr Stevenson's words or warnings, nor the explanations of other learned men, not these writings, not, I suspect, anything at all, is going to stop some new experimenter popping up to 'prove' to a credulous public that his case is real, and cannot be explained away by normal means; but you, who have come to understand the phenomenon of 'repression' should not find it at all difficult to understand what is really taking place, and know that the subject has already been done to death (sorry about the pun) and leave well alone. Try to come to a similar viewpoint to mine and consider all interest in the occult, supernatural, astrology, and even intense religious fervour as yet another presenting symptom of the individual's anxiety.

Considerably less mystical, but still really in the realms of the metaphysical, are subjects such as 'automatic writing' and the 'ideo-motor response' which you may have read about in books on hypnosis. Both techniques, to be wholly believable, require the subconscious to overrule the intellect. Well, from our studies we know that it not only can, but often does; but whether it will do so at the request of a hypnotist is a debatable point. In what is called the ideo-motor response the subject in hypnosis usually has it suggested to him that the first finger of his right hand is going to become immobile and rigid. In rather the same way as a person's eyelids can be made to 'stick' together, a skilful choice of words will ensure that the person is intellectually incapable of moving the finger. The subject is then told something to the effect that the finger is being linked to the subconscious mind and that any movement of the finger can only be effected by the subconscious; that the therapist proposes to ask questions of the subconscious and that the finger is to be lifted once for the answer yes, and twice for the answer no. There are as many variations of this theme as there are therapists, and likewise with 'automatic writing'; there are numerous techniques. Again the basic idea is that the subconscious mind shall be asked to dictate what the person writes down. Some techniques demand that the person closes his eyes with pen pressed to paper and simply lets the pen move at will.

I once saw a television programme about the use of hypnosis within the medical profession, and amongst the doctors put forward as experts was a one-time President of the British Society for Medical and Dental Hypnosis, who was using the hypnotic state to aid regression in an attempt to help a male patient overcome phonophobia or, as the learned doctor called it, voice paralysis. In the hypnotic state the subject could speak easily and naturally and the doctor was well pleased that after two years of treatment the patient was 'beginning to respond'.

It is sad, but unfortunately true, that the doctors who drift into hypnosis therapies are sometimes the misfits of their own profession and are motivated mostly by unconscious forces involving a need to externalize and identify. Whether that would be the case with this particular doctor I really would not like to say, but what did intrigue me (I was going to say amazed me, but nothing the medical profession does with hypnosis will ever amaze me) was the learned doctor's belief that he had so programmed his subject in the hypnotic state, that he would hear only the doctor's voice, and then only when speaking words addressed to the subject. The doctor quite happily chatted away to the observing spouse and commented, 'It's quite all right, he cannot hear us now.' Well, forgive them, they know not what they do!

Ask a somnambulist at the end of a hypnotic session what was said and what had taken place and he will say that he does not know and does not remember. It will be obvious that he is confused and believes he is telling the truth, and that he does not remember. Now prompt him with the odd word and you will find he is saying: 'Oh yes that's right, then you said . . .' and so on. Only a small amount of prompting will make his recall total. That learned surgeon turned hypnotist I was just talking about obviously had no conception of just that one fact. Most enlightened operating theatres have strict rules about what shall be said in the presence of a totally anaesthetized patient, especially relating to the patient's condition, as it is realized that the mind is still operating, and capable of assimilating harmful suggestions.

Every word of the foregoing should have convinced you that by no means do I consider the ideo-motor response infallible, nor yet do I take at face value what is written by a subject when an 'automatic writing' technique has been applied. I view what I am about to describe, not as the be all and end all of therapy, but just another lever to help loosen the repressions.

AUTO-WRITING TECHNIQUE

At some point during a session, when the client is snugly in hypnosis, I place a piece of plain paper and a ballpoint pen on my desk, and then tell the client that I am going to put my fingers on his forehead. While my fingers are on his forehead I want him to imagine something. I want him to imagine that it is possible for me to speak only to the subconscious of his mind. Then I lightly press two or three fingertips on his forehead and with some intensity of emotion in my voice I proceed as follows:

> The words that I now use are addressed only to the subconscious of your mind and all the time my fingers are on your forehead I am speaking only to the subconscious of your mind and it is a matter of complete indifference to both of us that you should be listening with your conscious intellect because the words are addressed only to the subconscious. When you sit up, when your eyes are open, on my desk you will see a piece of paper and a pen – and you will feel a need, an urge, a drive, a force, a compulsion to write something on the paper . . . to write words on the paper . . . and the thing that you will write, will be the thing that has troubled the subconscious, the thing that the subconscious has been at trouble to keep out of your thoughts – you will write it down, you will release it, own up and admit, but it is totally unnecessary for you to understand it yourself . . . if you want to think you have written something else, then you can, but what you will write will be the thing that has troubled the subconscious.

I would go through this twice, with intensity and a sort of

emotional charge to my voice in the hope that – What? You should be able to tell me by now. I am hoping that an idea will take root in the subconscious which must then of course be discharged in motor action by the individual. At this point I take my fingers from his forehead and without further comment about what I have done, I ask him to continue the process of free association of recall and, unless he dries up on me I do not speak again until I interrupt to terminate the hypnotic state near the end of the session. When he sits up I do not mention the paper and pen unless he is still avoiding it about three minutes later. Most clients will pick up the pen, comment that they do not know what to write, and then hastily write something down. I simply thank them, gather the paper up and fasten it to the back of their notes and once again wish them good-day as speedily as is polite, avoiding any discussion.

What have they written? Well, you can be fairly confident that it will be an indirect reference to the subconscious anxiety, although it is most unlikely that they will know that and it may well be difficult for you to see. I will give you an example. Our stuttering friend whom I have mentioned so often wrote: 'I'm going home now,' which, considering it was the end of the session, was apparently prompted by the intellect. However, at that person's next session he released a repressed memory of the incident where he had been indecently assaulted at the age of nine years, and the only words he had spoken to the assaulter were: 'I don't like this – I'm going home now'. A person may well write his own name, often her maiden name, if female, and this would infer a subconscious guilt about her own actions at some time. I use the technique purely because I have found it useful to help dislodge the repressed complex we are seeking. I know the person is perfectly capable of interfering intellectually with the process and do not set great store by the result. It is an aid, a weapon in your armoury, and that is all. But, just as any weapon is potentially lethal, so too, this technique can sometimes have amazing results and repercussions, and I have many times seen it be the determining factor of an analysis.

10. HYPNOSIS EXPLAINED

Now to fulfil a promise – to erase for ever from your mind any doubts you may have about your own ability to induce the hypnotic state.

First of all, do you understand all the earlier part of my writings? Say yes! . . . Well, in that case, you already know considerably more about hypnosis and its effects than does the average stage hypnotist. He knows what he does, he knows the effect he creates – but he has no idea why he does what he does (other than esoteric reasons) and no idea why what he does has those effects. So it transpires that you are already more knowledgeable in matters pertaining to hypnosis than is a professional hypnotist, who earns his living using, or rather misusing, the technique. You have also amazing factors working for you that the stage hypnotist has not. Many of his 'clients' are there for one reason only – to take the mickey out of him and play the fool. Your clients, or at least a high percentage, are paying you to hypnotize them.

Should you go to a professional photographer, you will get your photograph taken whether you approve of the resultant photograph or not; should you go to a professional artist, you will get your portrait painted – again, whether you like the resultant picture or not; should you go to a professional barber, you will get your hair cut whether you approve of the style he selects or not. Should you go to a professional hypnotist, you will get hypnotized whether you approve of the hypnotic state or not. The fact that hypnosis is the only one of the four examples which is intangible, which is abstract, does not lessen the validity of the analogy.

Pause in your thoughts for a moment upon my example of 'waking hypnosis', in Chapter 9. That accomplished dentist who so adeptly produced a psychosomatic effect understood what he was doing and why he was doing it. He knew he had to capture the person's attention. He knew he had to give a suggestion for the subconscious to act upon, and he knew there had to be an absence of counter-suggestion. Of course, it was easy for him – he had his dentist's white coat, his dentist's surgery, his dentist's chair; the person is there voluntarily; the person wants to believe what he is saying . . . Where is the difference between your clients and the dentist's? They want to be hypnotized – that is what they have come for. You are going to get their undivided attention. By inference you have already given a tremendously powerful suggestion without ever opening your mouth. Just by being there, just by being who you are, what you are, you have suggested that they are going to be hypnotized. Everybody expects a cobbler to cobble – and everybody expects a hypnotist to hypnotize people.

Hypnosis begins from the moment a person closes his eyes at the request or suggestion of the hypnotist. What the hypnotist actually says to the person, the way in which he says it, his voice control, his manner – of course they are all relevant, they are all contributing to the power of suggestion. But if a person goes to the consulting room of a professional hypnotist, he expects to be hypnotized – so, even if the hypnotist is somewhat inefficient, lacking the skills of his more professional counterparts, his clients still enter the hypnotic state – mostly because they expect to.

Should I ask a person to lie down on my consulting-room couch and say to them, 'I am going to hypnotize you – close your eyes now, please,' the person would naturally close his eyes. Hypnosis has now begun. Should I then read out the back page of the day's *Financial Times* in a soft, quiet tone, the client would deepen the state of hypnosis himself.

Most learned men of science who have investigated the hypnotic phenomenon in any depth have come to the same, or similar, conclusion – that hypnosis is achieved by the person himself as opposed to being achieved by the hypnotist. 'There is only auto - and not hetero - hypnosis': What the person expects to happen– does happen.

Perhaps, even after all my words so far, you persist in wanting to believe in magic, and feel inclined to draw my attention to a stage show you saw, where 'the people were made to do things in a trance, and a lot of them couldn't remember afterwards what had taken place'. Surely by now you have an understanding of the forces at work!

Let us now assemble one hundred people together and suggest to them that we are going to induce all one hundred into hypnosis. Let us make it clear to one and all that we are professional, that this is what we do for a livelihood and that as far as we are concerned what is going to take place is the most normal thing in the world, and that all one hundred will enter the hypnotic state, and find the state relaxing and enjoyable. We have not entertained the slightest doubt, we do not concede the slightest possibility of 'failure' – there is no such thing. All one hundred are going to enter the hypnotic state, and we say so. Although the degree of hypnosis will vary from person to person, they will enter the state – and we say so. We explain that the only persons who cannot be hypnotized are the mental defective and the inebriate, and we ask all such people to file quietly out – which of course still leaves us with all one hundred. We explain that there is no such thing as a hypnotized feeling and that most people do not feel that they have been hypnotized – but that, despite this, they will find it a pleasant and relaxing experience.

So to begin. With a large number, the easiest induction is from an 'eyes closed' start. (Hypnosis begins the moment the person closes his eyes at the request of the hypnotist.) So will everybody now please close their eyes, and please keep them closed all the time I am talking. Come on now, third row from the back, co-operate, close your eyes . . . thank you. Now, I want you all to keep your eyes closed all the time I am talking.

At this stage I do not propose to guide you, dear reader, through the exact wording of an induction because the actual words used are somewhat immaterial. What you are going to do is pass something, a suggestion, to the subconscious of their minds, and great minds of yesteryear (Coué and Baudoin) have laid down the requirements necessary:

1. Absence of counter-suggestion.
2. Intensity of attention.

We know that emotion will aid the process. We also have a clear understanding of Coué's law of reversed effort – I've told you already that you know more about hypnosis than the average professional hypnotist . . . believe me. Acquire belief – the final doubt to dispel.

We use words such as relax, sleep, calm, peace, deep, and so on, a lot in the hypnotic induction – and we acquire the technique of d-r-a-w-i-n-g such words out somewhat, as we are saying them. The words react upon the subconscious in a pacifying manner. Plenty of hypnotists say things such as 'You are going to fall into a deep, deep sleep.' Well, that is likely to produce a counter-suggestion internally: 'That's what he thinks.' So reword it: 'I want you to imagine that you are falling into a deep, deep sleep' – far less likely to invoke a counter-suggestion, and internal resistance.

Keep capturing each person's attention and focusing it by asking them to imagine various things . . . a pinprick of light at the end of a tunnel . . . darkness all around . . . a point of light in the darkness like a star . . . . Maintain a soothing, relaxing tone of voice and keep changing the point of focus you are asking them to imagine, and make sure those drawn-out sleeps, relaxers, etc., proliferate. After three minutes of your talk everybody is in hypnosis. Ask them now to imagine that their eyelids have stuck together, and stuck together so tightly that the more they try and pull them apart, the tighter they will stick together. Those few words so randomly linked together, are brimming over with what we have been learning. The very word 'try' is a suggestion by inference. What happens? Well, a few of the hundred 'fear' that it has happened, and Coué's law acts like Superglue. A few of the hundred had already relaxed so much that their eyes, behind closed lids (or sometimes partially closed lids) have inverted upwards. The up and down movement of the eyes is controlled by a muscle called the elevator expectorus, and this muscle gets its signals along the same nerve as the muscle controlling the eyelids. The nerve being already blocked (like a phone line engaged), the person cannot send the appropriate signal to the eyelids and Superglue takes over again. The message may partially transmit, causing the eyelids to flicker, but their eyes being turned upwards means that they cannot see anyway.

The vast majority of the hundred think to themselves: 'Well, I could open my eyes – but I won't bother.' The first stage of hypnosis is not called lethargic hypnosis without good reason. The person feels lethargic – their critical faculty is somewhat relaxed – they cannot be bothered to prove you wrong.

In the moments after your 'eyes stuck' suggestion, most of the hundred are thinking, 'I haven't heard the others move – they must all be hypnotized – everybody else's eyes must be stuck.' What they are really doing, of course, is giving themselves suggestions – auto-hypnosis – and consequently deepening the state.

Should you have 5000 people there, instead of your hundred, then one of the 5000 is likely going to open his eyes, look at you with pathetic attempts to conceal the triumph he's feeling, and by dint of all sorts of sign language, try and apologize to you for having such a strong mind that you could not master him. He is erroneously convinced that he was not hypnotized. Here I am really only quoting Sod's Law because I have no practical experience of such a happening. I can, in all honesty, state, that of the thousands and thousands of people I have asked to imagine their eyes 'stuck' together – whether there was one person in the room, ten people or five hundred people – nobody, but nobody . . . has ever opened their eyes at that point. I could count on one hand the number of people in that time who have, minutes afterwards, 'sneaked a quick peep' to make sure that they could. Hypnosis creates empathy – it really does.

Still have doubts? . . . Well, you are a pessimist aren't you. OK – latch on to this: I have told you that if you close your eyelids together, if you turn your eyes upwards in your head, you cannot open your eyelids without first lowering your eyes. Did you believe that? Well, try it. Try it now, I'll wait a moment while you do.

There now, I told you, didn't I. Well, utilize that effect – get your client to close his eyes, put your finger in the centre of his forehead, persuade him to look upwards with his eyes closed (you can easily see whether he does or not by the outline of his eyeballs against the lids). Persuade him to keep 'looking up at' your finger and say, 'I am going to count to three – when I get to three your eyelids will be stuck, and stuck tightly together. Stuck so tightly together that the more you try and pull them apart, the tighter and tighter they will stick together.' Now count to three and say, 'Go on, try; your eyelids are stuck together, keep looking at my finger from the inside even though your eyelids are stuck together.' Two chances, and two chances only:

1. He lowers his eyes, opens his eyelids and says 'Boo'.
2. He keeps his eyes up as requested, and consequently cannot open his eyelids.

In the case of (1), say 'Come on now, no cheating, close your eyes again and this time keep looking up at my finger.' In the case of (2) say, 'There you are – that's hypnosis.' From the start to finish of induction takes approximately twenty-five seconds. Now you can start to deepen the state by positively phrased suggestions. Should (1) persist a second time, say 'Ah! if you still want to experience the hypnotic state you are going to have to be a lot more co-operative', and then use a lengthier induction. The man's paranoid, of course – but that's no bar to the hypnotic state.

Generally speaking, the more intelligent the person the more readily he will accept hypnosis – intelligent as in bright and clever, that is, rather than intelligence as in academic qualifications. (We all know that the two do not, of necessity, go hand in hand – I have met university professors whose practical common sense left much to be desired.) The most responsive subjects of all are from the disciplined services – being used to accepting instructions and criticism they lack the egotistical resistance displayed by so many others.

As to why one person will go to the deeper states of hypnosis more easily than another, I confess I don't know. There – it's easy when you've said it. I don't know. Obviously it must have a certain amount to do with their 'suggestibility' – and suggestibility is yet another predisposition learned in those forming years. But there has to be more at work. Nobody yet has come up with an explanation, although investigations on the relationship of the different spheres of the brain have produced a wealth of interesting detail.

Once again, I shall airily dismiss the reasons as of no consequence anyway. I am not one who accepts that a person's suggestibility is increased by deepening the hypnotic state – his acceptance of the hypnotic state, to whatever depth, is amply sufficient for analysis to proceed. In the deeper states of hypnosis there would, in fact, be a minor barrier against analysis, not in favour of it, as the person would be too 'dreamy' to differentiate between fantasy and reality. In all the wealth of investigation and research carried out upon the hypnotic phenomenon nobody has ever shown that 'deepening' the state will enhance that person's ability to respond to post-hypnotic suggestion; in fact, the reverse has been proved. I mentioned in Chapter 7, during session three, a modern-day six-hour operation using hypno-anaesthesia in the USA. The subject was not in a somnambulistic state of hypnosis. The patient was in the lethargic state, and talked to the surgeon throughout the operation. The hypnotist involved (Myrna J. Morris) knew her stuff – knew that hypnosis does not, or rather should not, consist of getting the person to the deepest possible state that you can – perhaps even comatose – and then just piling suggestion upon suggestion. Hypnosis has to be learned. Yes, that's the right word – learned. The person has to learn hypnosis, and to learn something it is best, but not necessarily vital, to have a teacher.

Understand that, although abreactive experiences in the hypnotic phenomenon may bring about changes in a person, no amount of hypnosis alone will do so. Entering hypnosis is pleasant and relaxing – and that is it. Accepting a post-hypnotic suggestion from a hypnotist will temporarily programme your behaviour pattern – and that is it. Nothing else – no long-term changes, no magic.

I go a step further within my own beliefs and experience – I believe that a post-hypnotic suggestion needs the aid of the person's intellect to guide it, and the subject in deep states of hypnosis – who has lost his critical faculty – is less likely to respond well to post-hypnotic suggestion. So in my eyes, the 'brilliant' hypnotist whose expertise, manner, vocal ability and dynamism of character guide his clients to the deeper states, is not necessarily – in fact is probably not – a particularly good therapist.

Let me give you an example of what I mean. Somebody comes for help to stop smoking. Let us imagine that we go through a session with this errant smoker, giving suggestions about how easy he is going to find it to quit cigarettes: that when he puts a cigarette in his mouth the cigarette will taste awful; that the smell of cigarettes will revolt him. He forgot to mention – he smokes a pipe! He will spend most of the session thinking to himself, 'I'll stop the session in a moment and tell the therapist he's saying the wrong things because I smoke a pipe.' The lethargic state dictates that he won't stop the session, though. Your, or our imaginary therapist's, lack of research and error, doesn't matter two penny pieces. The client is just as likely – perhaps even slightly more likely – to stop smoking his pipe, as he would have been if your suggestions had been more accurately framed. What if he had been somnambulistic, though? Minus the intrusion of his own intellect, he would accept (or not accept, as the case may be) the suggestions verbatim – and stop smoking cigarettes. He would of course find the suggestion remarkably easy to act upon. To stop smoking cigarettes would be easy for him (I am being sarcastic, of course). The chances of him stopping smoking his pipe are somewhat remote, though with a proviso (and here goes my cynicism again) that having been to a hypnotist, having paid the hypnotist's fees, having been hypnotized – he's just likely to stop smoking anyway. Suggestion is a very, very powerful tool and suggestion does not, of necessity, have to be spoken.

Now I, as one who specifies evolution and not revolution, am going to say something which I consider rather profound, and apparently critical of hypnosis-orientated therapies. Before I do, though, I want to make it clear that I consider transcendental meditation, psycho-yoga, etc. – all the mind-relaxing therapies and techniques – to be one and the same thing, albeit with different names. I do not necessarily expect anyone to agree with me, but was rather hoping that your researches of the human mind from within these pages may well have led you to the same conclusion. Be that as it may, let me hark back for a moment to my mention of a TV programme about hypnosis and its application by a learned doctor to 'help' a man suffering with voice paralysis. In the same programme they showed a volunteer nurse being hypnotized by a psychiatrist. At a given point she was asked, whilst in the hypnotic state, to cast her mind back to a happy memory of childhood. Everybody seemed surprised that she promptly burst into tears over a very unhappy memory of childhood. I was not in the least bit surprised that she burst into tears. I know that the mind, in the hypnotic state, is hovering continually close to the release of subconscious anxiety.

Can you see where I am leading you yet, with this profound statement of mine? I do not see how I can turn the statement into a one-liner: in any case it would be a shame to spoil the habit of a lifetime – I will elaborate what I mean, though.

In the hypnotic state, with the subconscious surfacing like a bubble from the steadfastness of its ocean depths, the person – who is so relaxed and lethargic – is wide open to the release of subconscious anxiety. Wander off and leave him alone, still in the hypnotic state, for about half an hour, in the privacy of his own thoughts, and you will likely return to find him quietly weeping over an incident more than twenty years old. However, let us suppose that you, the professional hypnotist, did not know this, did not know that this was yet another phenomenon of the state, and the human mind. Let us further suppose that you are having your client attend each week for hypnosis and post-hypnotic suggestion therapy . . . Do you know, I think I can make it a one-liner after all – I believe you are making your client worse.

I think that any individual, who has been analysed out of his subconscious anxieties, and whose remaining repressions – such as they are – are very deep, would do well to experience the hypnotic state every day of his life. Unanalysed, I believe that regular acceptance of the hypnotic state (in whatever form – meditation, yoga, etc.) will cause subconscious anxieties to come closer to consciousness, and in consequence have a detrimental effect upon the psyche of the person. I know that what I am saying is contentious, but I believe it, and not without good evidence based on factual observations.

Within the very broad guidelines of the foregoing you should also be able to interpret why I do not think that legislation could ever effectively be brought to bear upon the subject of hypnosis and its derivatives. In order to pass a law, the legislature would first have to define hypnosis and what it is – and that alone should effectively hold them up for a few decades. Take it a step further and try and define psychotherapist, counsellor, psychologist and other such titles, and before you know it legislation could effectively turn your local neighbourhood priest into an unlicensed criminal. I know I faithfully promised to steer clear of religion, but I must just add that I believe that many people attending a high church service enter the hypnotic state during the service – unknowingly, of course. Perhaps just one more teeny sentence – I believe that the 'high priests' of yesteryear knew all that only too well, and that the chanting and ceremony were no idle choice of style. (By the way, I am not saying I do not think there will be legislation to do with hypnosis; what I am saying is that I do not think there will be effective legislation.)

When you have yourself experienced the truths which come out of your own analysis, when you finally stop believing in magic, when you only see hypnosis as a normal, ordinary, and immensely useful force – then, and only then, will you be able to harness the power for good that 'it' truly is.

Perhaps even after all that, after all my words and explanations you still doubt that you can do it? Oh ye of little faith! . . . All right then, you win . . . (In words of one syllable or so, here is how to 'hypnotize' someone.

1. Tell him you are a professional hypnotherapist and that you use hypnosis daily.
2. Tell him that you are going to hypnotize him.
3. Say, 'Fine, just close your eyes and I will begin. Keep your eyes closed all the time I am talking and just relax. Just relax. Let all your muscles just sag limply and relax. Imagine yourself looking upwards into darkness. Just imagine yourself looking upwards in darkness, imagine a tiny pinprick of light in that darkness . . .'.

Continue with that sort of dialogue for three minutes – that's it – he is hypnotized – you've done it.

There are obviously an enormous number of induction procedures which can be used, and enough other writers have committed them to print to save me the trouble. It takes a trained eye, however, actually to observe the hypnotic state. When your eyes are sufficiently well trained you will be able to see the signs. Meanwhile, just accept that the person is hypnotized. Should you ever doubt it then you will feel remarkably foolish when you later have become expert enough to recognize the signs. You will then realize that when you thought you had failed, you had not. The stages 1–3 I have just listed will hypnotize anyone, except for a mental defective or an inebriate – it is only the degree of hypnosis which will vary.

THE SIGNS OF HYPNOSIS

What of these signs which it takes such experienced eyes to detect? At long last, is this to be the magical factor? I am afraid not. Again it is all rather ordinary.

1. A significant number of people will have an observable facial flush as they enter hypnosis which will remain while hypnosis remains.
2. A significant number of people will experience a flickering of the eyelids as they enter the hypnotic state. The flickering usually subsides within a second or so – but for some the flickering would continue for 10, 15, 20 seconds or so.
3. A significant number of people will experience an inversion of the eyes as they enter the hypnotic state – the eyeballs will roll upwards behind their closed lids. Occasionally that will cause their lids to part by about an eighth of an inch, thus displaying the whites of their eyes.
4. A small number of people will experience a drooping of the eyelids as they enter the hypnotic state, so that their eyelids droop to a three-quarter-closed position. Should you have started hypnosis on these people with their eyes closed, then their eyes will part slightly as they enter the hypnotic state, then staying drooped in that three-quarter-closed position. They can see through the open lids but their field of vision is restricted and they seldom move their eyes.
5. A small number of people will experience a tingling sensation on the surface of the skin, particularly on the face, and this will often cause them to scratch their face.
6. A small number of people will keep making facial grimaces throughout the session – distorting their features into quite unpleasant shapes. This is an involuntary action and they would usually not be aware of it.
7. A significant number of people would experience total muscular relaxation progressively throughout the session. So, if seated, the head would gradually fall

forward or to one side, the mouth would gape slightly, all their features would sag into repose.

8. A moderate number of people would experience partially the catatonic state during the hypnotic experience in that some (occasionally all) of their muscles would become rigid and stiff. It is observable if it affects the hands, which it often does – giving them a claw-like appearance.
9. A very small number of people would go somnambulistic in the session and demonstrate all the signs of sleep.
10. A tiny, tiny number of people will go so somnambulistic that they verge on comatose and will not respond to your 'wake up' suggestions (I will be coming back to this in due course).
11. A significant number will experience a heaviness and deadness in their limbs throughout the session. This is only becomes observable if you see them struggling to lift one leg off the other, or such.
12. A significant number of people will experience a lightness of limbs, and a vague floating sensation throughout the session – this is not observable.
13. A modest number of people will experience a vague disjointed sort of feeling during the session, as though they were not quite sure that their limbs are lying exactly where they left them – again this is not observable.
14. A small number of people will experience a fast falling sensation very briefly in the session. This will give them a visible 'jolt'.
15. A very significant number of people will experience a time distortion to a factor of between two, and two and a half times, through the session, i.e. their estimate of time elapsed during a fifty-minute session would be twenty minutes. This of course can be checked upon.
16. A very small number of people would experience a totally opposite time distortion so their estimate was 'over two hours'. This too can be checked.
17. A small number of people will experience a discharge of emotion (usually tears) during the session with no apparent intellectual explanation. Depending upon the emotion concerned it may be observable.
18. A very small number of people will involuntarily open

their eyes about half-way through the session. Normally they would close them again within a few seconds. Their gaze would have been rather blank. Should their eyes remain open their gaze will remain blank.

19. Most people will experience dilation of the eye pupils throughout the session. This would not normally be observable due to their closed lids.
20. A small number of people will experience a tingling sensation akin to 'pins and needles' usually in their nether regions. This too is not observable.
21. A significantly large number of people will be well content to remain where they are at session end and will often say so: 'I could stay here for the rest of the day.'
22. A moderate number of people will respond visibly to suggestions relating to change in temperature, unusual smells, unpleasant or pleasant taste, etc.
23. A moderate number of people will 'swallow' abnormally often as they enter the hypnotic state.
24. A small number of people will experience a sensual feeling, perhaps resulting in sexual arousal, throughout the session.
25. Many juveniles will experience that same sensual feeling quite sharply. In the juvenile male it would be observable as a series of rapid movements of the penis, almost a 'threshing' – presumably an equal number of juvenile females experience a similar, but unobservable, phenomenon.
26. A moderate number of people will experience cramp or other muscular rigidity in the hands or legs which persists after the session for a while – usually only minutes.
27. Most people will experience a tiny, split second, of 'realization' or 'understanding' as they leave the hypnotic state. At the split second the eyes open, for one tiny instant of time . . . something, an unknown something . . . is different. A split second later . . . it is just as normal as I told you it always was.
28. Most people's respiration and heart rate will slow well down.
29. Most people's brain-wave cycle will slow down. This of course is not observable (without an alpha brain-wave meter).

30. Most people's electrical resistance of the skin surface will drop by 20 per cent. Again not observable without an extremely accurate meter (or bio-rhythm counter).
31. Most people's hearing will improve throughout the duration of the session. Again, this takes instruments to check, but what usually happens is that the normally placid side of the person's hearing is increased to match the ability of the dominant side (right-handed – left ear; left-handed – right ear).
32. Well, I think I have listed enough, because if I continue I am going to get awfully technical. Suffice it to say that the two known branches of the autonomic nervous system – the sympathetic and the parasympathetic – have, according to some scientists, got further subdivisions, namely the endophinergic and the endoloxonergic. Hypnosis does, or rather would appear to, have effects upon those areas.

I had better go back to point number 10 because it can happen – in fact, does happen. Sometimes, just occasionally, a really anxious 'bag of nerves' finds the hypnotic phenomenon so totally relaxing – it is the first time he has really relaxed for years .... Sometimes, just sometimes, a natural somnambulist accepts the hypnotic state so readily; sometimes, again only sometimes, a Valium taker, or other drug taker, accepts the hypnotic state so readily; occasionally a very heavy drinker accepts the state so readily – in one of these instances you just might find that the end of the session . . . just isn't the end of the session.

My normal (I always feel tempted to put that word in inverted commas every time I use it) method of bringing a session to a close is to say, 'And now, I would like you in your own thoughts, not out loud, only in your own thoughts, I would like you to count slowly up to five – and when you get to five just to open your eyes again, please.' Oh! there's point number 33 for my list – most people will take a while, well over five seconds, to count to five! However, what about this 'just occasionally' I was talking about, when thirty seconds later there has been no response to your request. No problem, usually – you just say, 'Right, we'll both count to five. When I get to five you will be wide awake. One – waking up now, two

– rising up, three – getting bright now, four – feeling bright, waking up, five – open your eyes, open your eyes.' But, just occasionally, once in a blue moon – still no response. OK – go through it again, brighter and livelier and louder. Still no response? Well, now – to be honest, you've got a bit of a problem on your hands, particularly if you have a busy schedule the rest of the day. If you haven't a busy schedule, well, just let him get on with it, it is doing him a world of good anyway. Every fifteen minutes or so go through a fairly loud 'wake up' procedure. Sooner or later he will. (He'll still swear he was never hypnotized, mind you – there is no such thing as a hypnotized feeling.) But what if you do have a busy schedule, what if you need to get rid of him? How exactly do you break the state? To be honest, with the greatest of difficulty! Try holding his eyelids open and going through your 'wake up' count. Try blowing on the side of his face between each number of the count. Try lifting his arm, unless it is rigid, and letting it drop with each count. Try – but be ready to get quickly out of the way – saying the one word 'Danger' very quietly in his ear. That, by the way, is a drastic, last-resort step, and may well produce an almost primaeval response.

I have a better idea – just hope it never happens to you and your client. Be assured, the person can come to no harm, and other than inconvenience value, it doesn't matter one jot. Laugh about it. Use that 'unusualness' I said was necessary to the character of an analyst.

Having listed all those observable, and non-observable phenomena of the hypnotic state, I should hate to think that you had the idea that any one client would demonstrate all, or indeed, any one of the phenomena. There is another, an intangible, an indescribable, about the hypnotic state – when you've seen it often enough you can recognize it. Way back, I used the analogy of electricity: you can't see it, you can't hear it, you can't smell it, you can't taste it – but it can't half bite, and you just 'know' it's there; you don't have to get hold of the bare wires to find out. You will find you become the same with hypnosis – you just know that it is there.

Well, there you are, I promised to dispel your doubts about your abilities as a hypnotist – and so I have. You have finally acquired that belief – the final doubt to dispel.

GO AND DO IT

You need practice now to develop your own personal technique, so hypnotize everyone you meet. Milkman, postman, local shop proprietor, landlord of your local pub, wife, husband, children, colleagues, friends, acquaintances – anyone who will let you. Never, but never, commence an induction unless you intend to take it to a conclusion. Years ago, a female subject pleaded with me to demonstrate hypnosis to her in a social situation. Somewhat foolishly I complied, but, as she felt herself 'going' she fought it and said, 'No, stop it. I've changed my mind,' and desperately tried to resist the onset of the state. I applied what is called the 'eye-to-eye fascination method' where you simply 'capture' the subject's gaze with yours and just continue your induction talk. She mentally fought about as hard as anybody before or since, but – the onset of the state is inevitable, provided you know the outcome, and I did, and I do. She could not avert her gaze – the 'fascination effect', like a snake with its prey, is a very powerful effect. She verbally pleaded, 'Please don't hypnotize me' over and over again. Coué's law held her inexorably in its grasp, until, of course – she entered the hypnotic state. Later, when I asked her to release the state, she was most reluctant to do so, and heaped superlatives upon what a nice feeling it had been. Nowadays, I probably would never allow that situation to arise; but, if I did, if I commenced an induction, then I would always carry it through to a conclusion.

You will find it impossible to keep hypnosis and therapy entirely separate from your private life. Friends and acquaintances will have a consuming curiosity upon the subject. I can only say that every single time I have allowed myself to be drawn, I have regretted it – and vowed that it would be the very last time. With the inevitability of fate, I get drawn again; but these days it really is very, very rarely. I try to practise as I preach and content myself with being right – parrying all questions, challenges, insinuations, and the like, with a jocular reply. Occasionally though – well, you wouldn't be human – the last time this worm turned was at a party at a friend's house. A guy there was being just a bit of a pain, and I'd stood, with good-humoured tolerance, just about every insult along the lines of being a practitioner of the black arts, that anyone should be asked to stand. I listened to it all – how no one would ever hypnotize him, no member of his family would ever – etc., etc. Now, over the years, one thing I have learnt is to recognize a responsive subject; and I had already mentally noted that his wife was potentially a very responsive subject. I turned to her, caught her eyes with mine, and said, 'Cross the fingers of your right hand. The first and forefinger of your right hand – cross them. (She did.) I am going to count to three – when I get to three you will feel your fingers stick tightly together. When I get to three, the harder you try to uncross your fingers the tighter they will stick together' – all this with her gaze firmly held. Then I theatrically counted to three – her fingers stuck (of course) and then I said, 'You are now in hypnosis. In a moment your eyes will close and you will go deeply to sleep, but your body will remain rigid, and you will stay standing exactly where you are.' She did (of course). Then I turned back to the husband and said, 'You see – it's not all that difficult after all – excuse me, there's someone I must talk to.' I walked off, to his intense consternaton and with him at my heels pleading for the restoration of his wife. I let him worry about it for about five full minutes with the wife as still as a statue and then went and asked her to release the state. She did (of course) and said what a lovely euphoric feeling it had been, and how much she was enjoying the party. I never did get around to asking her husband whether he enjoyed the party, though.

I don't say I acted very professionally, or all that ethically, but we are all very fallible human beings, aren't we. I would add a self-justification too. If I had thought for one moment that his wife would have been the least upset by it then I would not have done it. I might take the odd liberty or two with hypnosis, but I would never consciously abuse its use.

Hopefully not having destroyed my credibility in your eyes, I will just touch on another point. You can hypnotize people. It is very easy. So, of course, you can hypnotize yourself. Again, it is easy. Enough other people have written clear enough instructions for me to save my ink. But you know a bit more than they do now – because you know what effects to expect and, more importantly, not to expect. You know that with auto- or hetero- suggestion you must avoid the negative like the plague, or you risk Coué's retribution. You know enough to be able to 'programme yourself' to be whatever you want to be. Well – why not a first-class analyst, therapist and hypnotist? Use self-hypnosis and auto-suggestion to aid yourself, to become expert; or more expert than you already are.

11.
SOME TECHNICAL DIFFICULTIES AND DREAMS

I promised to touch on some of the more technical difficulties of analysis, as opposed to the more general difficulties which I have outlined previously. To introduce the subject I want first of all to mention dreams and their interpretation. By now, with the insight you should have acquired, dreams should have less of their mysteries concealed. When you have a decade or so to spare, wade your way through Freud's masterpiece *The Interpretation of Dreams*, which caused the great man himself to comment that 'insight such as this falls to one's lot but once in a lifetime'. I should think he would be awfully disappointed if he knew the exact number of people who have since acquired similar insight by a perusal of his writings, because I bet you would not need two hands to count them on.

Now, although I would not claim to be an expert, I do use dream interpretation in my work. With a high percentage of clients I include, towards the end of the first session, a post-hypnotic suggestion: 'The tensions in your mind will be relieved at night in your dreams – and you will remember your dreams . . . no matter they do not make sense . . . you will remember your dreams and write them down, please. You will remember and write down your dreams.' One could at that point include a suggestion to 'bring them to me', which of course would serve a twofold purpose. Perhaps your mind is not as devious as mine. . . yet! Can you see that if you do include those last four words, you have given the person a post-hypnotic suggestion to come back for session two? . . . or at least to come back. Bit naughty that, isn't it? Perhaps you will have to be more devious still, because if the client thought, 'He's trying to make sure I come back,' then that is one client you would probably never see again. Should the supposed suggestion take root in the subconscious – then of course it will ensure his return.

When a client dutifully brings me in his dreams, I do not comment upon them. I fasten them to his notes, and read them in his absence. I will interpret them, and I will keep my version of their interpretation to myself. I will not discuss them with the client.

As the analysis proceeds, you will see the subject matter of the dreams, albeit symbolic, appearing in the recall of the client. I mentioned you will normally come to intellectual insight into your client's problem long before he does – well, his dreams, and their interpretation, should confirm (again, to you) that your insight is correct . . . and . . . if the analysis begins to founder you can gently 'lead him' back on course. How? Well, you await a pause, and then you remind him of three or four things he has already related (carefully choosing three or four which are 'near misses' for what you have in mind) and then to say the very next thing that comes into his thoughts. It is like putting him back on the railway track but without setting the points. He dictates the direction of travel.

Amongst thousands of dream interpretations I have made, two stick in my mind, and they are worth the telling.

I once, very casually, said to a lady client that most dreams are wish-fulfilments. Next week she stormed into my consulting rooms at session time like a juggernaut, clutching a written-out dream in her hot little fist. 'Are you going to tell me I wish my husband dead?' says she, thrusting the paper in my hands. The dream concerned her husband. In the dream he'd traded his car for a tatty old banger full of rust and holes . . . he'd painted the windscreen black, on the inside and the outside . . . he'd dragged her roughly by the wrist and thrust her in the passenger seat . . . he'd roared off down the road like a lunatic . . . he'd gone straight across a junction, crashed into a lorry and he'd been killed stone dead – with blood everywhere. In the circumstances I had no real alternative but to offer her an interpretation. I made it in the form of question and answer.

Q: Has your husband just bought a new car he's proud of?
A: Fairly recently – it's the pride of his life.
Q: What are the chances of him trading it in for a 'tatty old

banger full of rust'?

A: Nil.

Q: If he did – what are the chances of him painting the windscreen black?

A: Well, he wouldn't, would he?

Q: What are the chances of him dragging you roughly by the wrist and thrusting you into the car?

A: He wouldn't dare.

Q: What are the chances of him driving like a maniac?

A: He is a most careful driver.

There! say I. It turns out it is a wish-fulfilment dream after all. A wish not to be involved in an accident. If your husband satisfies the conditions of the dream he will have an accident and be killed; if he doesn't – he won't. 'Well, you devious bastard,' she said in a jocular tone. 'No, lady,' say I, 'You're the one who had the dream.' I did not elaborate that I consider there is a deeper, far more symbolic, interpretation to be put upon the dream, concerning the fears and fantasies of youth. Can you see it?

Story two, that sticks in my mind, was at a Christmas party when I heard a female voice behind me saying, 'I want to be introduced to him.' I glanced round the pilot, solicitor and other professional people present and thought, 'Here we go again!' Minutes later – there she was. The upshot was that she insisted on telling me a repeating dream that gave her nightmares twice a week and had done for years. I tried to palm her off with a visiting card, I joked that 'nobody else was working, it's Xmas', I warned her that telling me her dreams was revealing the most intimate of her thoughts; but, would she be put off? – no, she wouldn't. Eventually I said, 'OK, but if you tell me the dream so people hear, I will tell you my interpretation – equally out loud.' She was delighted (then) and proceeded to recount the dream, which consisted of her going back to her old house, only to find all the lights on, and a sports car outside. She went in through the open door, and it was obvious the house had been burgled. She ran round the house looking and when she got back to the bottom of the stairs, she found her cat lying there, split wide open and pouring blood. The cat had been white but it gradually turned black. End of dream.

So I interpreted. I explained that when people dream of a house, they are quite often, certainly not always, dreaming of themselves, the organism as a whole – so, the upstairs windows would be the eyes, and so on. I explained that to dream of your old house would often mean to dream of your body – as it used to be. (She was still quite intrigued – at this stage.)

Let us suppose, I said, that such an interpretation was correct, that you were dreaming of your body as it used to be. But it was 'burgled', it was 'broken into' – by a fellow in a sports car – and the lights were on when he did it. I bet somebody else can interpret that, I said, without my help. Let's move on: 'at the bottom of the stairs' the cat cut in half. Give me another word for cat – try 'pussy' – cut in half, pouring blood? Changing from virginal white – obvious surely . . and then I finished in a flurry. 'I suspect that you have been dreaming about the first time you had sex, with a fellow in a sports car; it took place in a well-illuminated spot, and that, minus your virginity, you lost a fair bit of blood . . . Am I right?' Exit one dreamer hurriedly to the ladies'. However, to her credit, she came back fairly quickly, having recovered her composure and said that it was amazingly accurate, and that she somehow 'knew' that the interpretation was correct. I met her a few months later (accidentally – honest) and she confided that she had never had the dream since. That is, of course, the confirmation that my interpretation was correct. I will leave dreams at that, otherwise I could go on for ever and probably bore you to tears.

Let me get back to difficulties. One you have to nip in the bud at its onset is intellectualization. Let me try and illustrate.

A client is lying as good as gold in lethargic hypnosis at session two. You say, '. . . And now I want you to tell me what you find yourself thinking about.' Let's suppose the client has just had a fleeting recall of one time when he was sat at the dinner table . . . Mum came in . . . gave him a bang around the head and told him to take his elbows off the table. The client should, of course, say, 'I am remembering being at the dinner table. When I was about ten, my mum came in and gave me a belt round the back of the head for having my elbows on the table. I was very upset.' That's what the client should say, but sometimes instead: 'I'm just remembering my old mum and how good she usually was to us.' 'Can you tell me what you were thinking of that has made you make that comment?' 'Just my old mum. She was a good mum! . . .' 'Yes, but what did you recall that has made you say that?' 'Well, nothing really. I don't want you to get the wrong idea about my mum. She was a good mum.' 'Will you please tell me what it is you recalled that has brought this whole conversation?' 'You'll think she was a bad mum. It's nothing, really it isn't.' 'Will you please tell me what you'd thought of?' 'Well, I'm remembering being at the dinner table . . .' etc.

Your persistence finally pays off, and he tells verbatim. The analysis must consist of the 'psychological experiences' of the past. The person has 'intellectualized' his problem for thirty years before he came to you; to continue applying intellect to the problem will serve no purpose at all, and he mustn't be allowed to. 'Most people do not know what they want – those who do know . . . should give it to them.' No doctor ever asks his patient whether he thinks he should have Valium or perhaps Ativan. He prescribes what he knows to be correct. Likewise, you should make sure the analysis proceeds the way you want it to – always trying not to influence the direction, though.

Another difficulty to overcome is silence! Silence is about the biggest difficulty of all. In analysis, a mere five seconds of silence is too much. The client must be cajoled into relating whatever comes into his thoughts, and his thoughts are almost never empty. Should he just have a 'picture' of his dining room in his thoughts, he should be cajoled into saying so, and not allowed to stay silent waiting for a memory.

Counter all the objections with, 'That's all right, just relax and tell me whatever you think about.' When he says that there are hundreds of thoughts crowding in his mind, just say, 'Relax, and tell me the first thing you think about.' When he says his thoughts are blank, just say, 'Relax, and tell me the first thing you think about.' All the time you are aiming to get your client just to say out loud whatever occurs to him. It is not much to ask really – not like asking him to swim the Atlantic; but sometimes I think the latter would be easier.

There is the time between sessions, too. One has to allow at least five days' interval and no more than, say, an eight- or nine-day interval, otherwise the process is interfered with.

During that time, the client is in the presence of the biggest enemy of all – relatives. What a pain relatives and friends are, with their 'well-meaning', 'expert', self-satisfied opinions – if only they'd keep their interfering noses out.

Just for a moment I want you to imagine that you were to go to your closest relative – no, make that your mother. Imagine going to your mother, and telling her that you were going to an analyst to be cured of – whatever. Imagine telling your mum that the analyst was going to search your childhood for the cause of the disorder. Do you think he would get her blessing and approval? Tell you what – if you have still got a mum, try it, and see what happens. I'll bet you she scores the idea nought out of a hundred. Her subconscious fear, and conscious worry, will be that her 'sins' and failings as a mother will all be revealed. She will join that long line of people who think you should 'shake yourself out of it'. ('Not that I'm inferring you are other than perfect, of course') and she will likely heap scorn and doubt upon analysis as a therapy.

If the truth was known, people like the 'status quo', and friends and relatives have got used to the 'neurotic' one being the way he is; and if that person's recovery means an interference in their closeted little lifestyle, well . . . .

What of the client who just won't see his enlightenment when it's staring him in the face? I mean the one who has had six sessions or so and whose every recollection is a blatantly close, but indirect, reference to the complex you just know you are in search of. Often you will notice that when a particular memory is very close to what you 'know' is concealed, his next recollection will be of an incident where he got a bang on his head. Whenever a client produces a recollection of a bang on the head, however he got it, always recap the preceding recollection out loud for him, and then again ask him to say the next thing that comes into his thoughts. Usually, but of course not always, the person recounting an incident of a bang on the head is really symbolically saying, 'I don't remember something to do with that last memory.' (It will save you a lot of hassle if you simply believe what I've just written now because you will, later, when you have seen it happen a few hundred times.) There comes a stage with this type of client – who just won't face himself and his hang-ups – when you might just as well 'slap him across the face with it' – say about session eight or nine. By then your intellectual insight to the cause of his problem should be total, and if you have a couple of dreams from him that confirms it – OK break the rules. It does not matter now, anyway – it's make or break. Verbally 'accuse' him of the complex you have in mind and ask him to say the next thing that comes into his thoughts. Do it again, and again; if your onslaught gets to him, he'll 'see' it for himself – intellectually, but far more importantly – emotionally. Should he remain impervious to your barrage, then he's L.M.F. (army expression - 'lacking moral fibre'), he's beyond the reaches of analysis: send him back to a drug-orientated therapy.

Probably the most frustrating of all difficulties for the analyst is when the client has arrived at the 'abstract' stage and gone through a sequence of recollections in a vague form, quoting the usual 'It's as though I was seeing it on film'; 'It's imagination, I'm sure'; 'I can't seem to think of anything else' – having arrived at this stage and just refusing to go beyond it. The subconscious resistance is so total and the conscious objections so strong he sticks at that. When he returns for the next session he has decided that 'it' couldn't be true . . . not of him . . . he would never have done anything 'like that' . . . it must have all been imagination . . . 'I probably invented it just to please you' . . . Should that attitude prevail for a couple of sessions it can be the most frustrating of technical problems to overcome. These days I would not even bother to help the person try to overcome it; I would discharge him from analysis. Time, and the dissolution of transference, will do the rest. His intellect will remain puzzled to why he had produced such an imaginary sequence, and sooner or later, it will come to him: he will arrive at a sense of inner conviction of the validity of the material. Whether it is later, rather than sooner, is of small account; his nervous disorder didn't exactly arrive yesterday; it is not a 'squared off' problem, it is a growing, maturing thing, as he himself is.

So: OK, there are a few problems connected with analysis using hypnosis. So! Whoever got to be happy and contented in life without overcoming a few problems? Whoever got to be rich and famous, without overcoming thousands of problems? So! There are a few problems connected with analysis – that's good, that's great, that's terrific – we just set to and overcome those problems. We can, we will, and we're going to.

All in all it is just about time for you to grab a volunteer for analysis. You know what to do, you know why you would be doing it. You know how you would be doing it, and you know – or think you know – the merit to be obtained for the person you do it for. *Unless, of course, you'd like to make that first volunteer yourself.*

12.
TWO CASE HISTORIES

Armed with your new-found enlightenment, read through the following two sets of case notes of mine which, at one time or another, have been published in professional journals, and I wouldn't mind betting that you understand what took place to effect the cures, whereas I know full well that my previous readers hadn't got much of a clue as to what I was talking about.

CASE ONE
ALL'S WELL IN THE END or THE CASE OF THE PATIENT WIFE

We should be immune to surprises, but the well-built, expensively dressed gentleman who consulted me – bearing all the outward signs of a man who has made a success of forty-plus years – nevertheless managed to lift at least one of my eyebrows (slightly, and of course, imperceptibly) when, in cultured tones he informed me that, for the previous seventeen years he had been attempting to consummate his marriage – with a singular lack of success.

Classically his 'executive organ of sexuality' demonstrated all the signs of readiness until the moment approached for penetration, when, like most other cases of psychical impotence, he experienced a sinking sensation both physically and psychologically.

He confided that over the seventeen-year period he had spent some £3500 plus on private medical fees in an attempt to alleviate the condition, as well as suffering every indignity the NHS and sexual dysfunction units had heaped upon him. At one time the pills and potions had left him feeling so fit and elated he was jumping five-bar gates before breakfast – but his other hurdle remained uncrossed.

When we got down to the analytical process his first recollection was of his mother, breast-feeding his younger sister; then, as the memories unwound, he recalled fright – at the early sight of a woman's genitals; he remembered fear – and puzzlement, at blood on the toilet seat; he recalled being indecently assaulted by a 'dirty old man'; he vividly remembered wetting himself – and being told if it happened again 'it' would be cut off.

The case was remarkable only for its ease of success. These random memories, all vaguely linked to the aforesaid complexes, in just four sessions, led to the release of a repression of the mind, which took the following form.

Through the haze he saw himself at the glass door of their lounge at about the age of four. The pictures then started to come clearer and he saw his mother, and a man, lying together on the settee. Their movements intrigued him, and he could recall thinking that it would be fun to ask Mummy afterwards if he could play the same game with her as the man. When the man withdrew and knelt up, he saw the man's penis and recalled thinking that it was only a larger version of his own and so he would be able to play the game all right. He then, in his mind, went into the room to speak to the errant pair – much to their consternation. Then there was a lot of hurried rearrangement of clothing, and he was coerced 'never to tell' – that when Daddy came back 'it was to be their secret'.

At this stage all would have perhaps been well. The boy loved his mum and liked the man and although the incident had been interesting it had by no means made a profound impression. He quite liked the idea of keeping a secret with those of whom he was so fond – after all, Dad was a rather vague memory of someone who'd gone away.

What led to the repression and the subsequent neurosis was a later action of the man. He later that day got the boy in his bedroom, and threatened what he would do if ever the boy told. To reinforce his threats he took out a knife and threatened to cut off the boy's penis if ever one word left his lips. He even took out the lad's penis and demonstrated a cutting action. This, of course, produced an agonizing fear in the boy which led to the memory being lost in repression

I am sure that you, dear reader, need no further explanation of the case, which was, of course, resolved from that moment on. A few days later I had a message on my answer-phone service (which I have taped for my memoirs). After introducing himself my client said, 'Mr French, after last night I felt I must ring and – thank you very much – thank you very much – thank you very much. I'm sure you will know what I mean'. I think I did, do you?

Post-Case Comment

When the memory to do with his mother was subconscious it was having a devastating effect upon his psyche. The bringing to intellectual consciousness of the memory caused that effect to cease. His maturity now came to his rescue: within a very short while the memory matured so he began to feel that he had always known about his mother and the man, which, of course, subconsciously, he always had. When the memory matured it became a matter of indifference to him. He blamed only himself for the whole misadventure – after all he had wanted to do 'rude things' to Mummy. His guilt and his fears were released by analysis and he was freed of them. Aha! I know a little postscript to this particular case. He made the mistake of telling his wife what had come out in analysis. Now, to her, it was not a thirty-odd-year-old memory revived, it was a brand new revelation. Her first words? – 'Well, the sanctimonious old cow – that's the last time she ever sets foot in this house.' No amount of explanation would suffice. She had made her assessment. The mother's fornication with the man was the cause of those seventeen long years of frustration, and that was that. The marriage came nearer to foundering over that issue to do with his mother, than ever it did through his previously 'floppy penis'. Some things just cannot be explained – they have to be lived through.

CASE TWO
DECISIONS – ALL THE TIME DECISIONS

Freud would have wallowed in this analysis: Single girl, aged 24 years who consulted with insomnia, migraines and an anxiety state. These were the problems which she brought to me, but she soon revealed an extra 'problem' which is probably the clearest demonstration possible of the link between anxiety and sexuality.

The girl explained that, whenever she was confronted with a decision to take, then if she decided quickly, all was well, but – if she dithered, and felt the least anxious about the decision – even something as trivial as a choice between two dresses to purchase – then she would come to an immediate, and involuntary, sexual climax.

She had been aware of this phenomenon from the age of about eight years, when, if confronted with anxiety or decision, she had experienced what she came to know as one of her 'nice moments'. This was the nickname she and her mother had given to the feeling she had described as like a hot flush in her tummy, which gripped her whenever the anxiety arose. After puberty the feeling had changed to become a total orgasm. Predictably, she was unable to experience such a climax through the sexual act.

Her analysis proceeded fairly smoothly, and revealed, amongst other things, an amazing recollection of herself falling from a nine-storey window at the age of three – her life being saved by a bush planted only hours previously in an otherwise paved courtyard.

The falling sensation was abreacted; likewise, too, the sensations created by a twice-daily warm oil massage on her tender young bottom – and her intense hatred of the nurse administering this massage – were recalled most vividly.

Her adult dreams nearly always took the form of sexual fantasies of two women and one man and the analysis quickly revealed the Oedipal origination. The most significant point had been the break-up of the parent's marriage when she had been six or seven years old. She had been presented with an ultimatum: to choose which of the two parents she wanted to live with, the parents having agreed in their 'wisdom' to let the little girl's decision be the deciding factor.

Happily the analysis proceeded to a satisfactory conclusion, and her 'nice moments' now take place at the appropriate moment of sexuality. The insomnia, migraines and anxiety have ceased. Most interestingly: she has since found herself exchanging all her old friends for a complete new circle of acquaintances, as her previous friendships were mostly of the 'gay' fraternity. Her inability to make decisions had at its origin an unconscious conflict regarding her choice of sexual object, and unknown to herself, she had been 'playing safe'.

Post-Case Comment

The lady in question is now happily married.

INDEX